W0254381

Gut efficiency; the key ingredient in pig and poultry production

Gut efficiency; the key ingredient in pig and poultry production

Elevating animal performance and health

edited by:

J.A. Taylor-Pickard

P. Spring

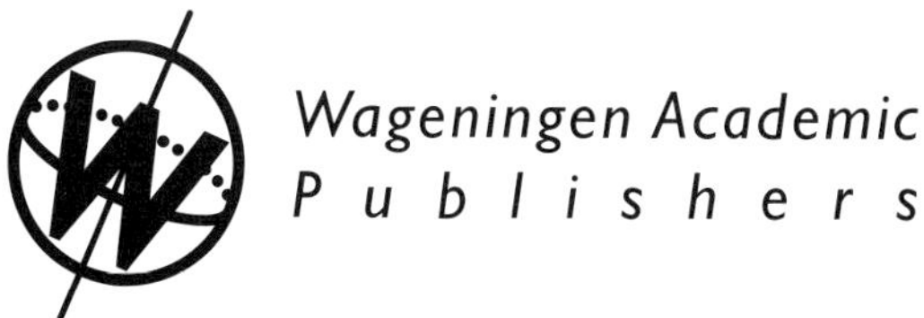

ISBN: 978-90-8686-060-9

First published, 2008

Wageningen Academic Publishers
The Netherlands, 2008

Contents

How past experience can dictate future developments in the pork industry: a global perspective

Roger Campbell
Pork CRC, P.O. Box 466, Willaston SA 5118, Australia

1. Introduction

The drivers of profit in pork production have always been and remain the price received for the product and the cost of feed. Consequently, factors that affect the demand for pork and the price of grain will generally have the biggest impact on the business of producing pork. In this respect we owe a lot to the plant breeders who have delivered consistent improvements in yields and to agronomists who have generally enabled the potential offered by new grain varieties to be exploited. Price is a different matter and is affected by changes in both domestic and global demand for pork and competing meats, especially beef and chicken. In the time I have been involved in the pork industry price has always been difficult to predict, and until recently was generally determined by the market place although many producers now attempt to remove some of the risk on the price side through supply contracts with packers and to a lesser extent through the future markets. There has been no doubt that the 'quality' of pork has improved over time with the changes being driven by the processing industry in response to retailer and consumer demands. Indeed, in terms of pork quality there really isn't much that isn't known, and more importantly, most of the 'recommendations' for improving quality have been implemented at the production and processor levels. The next step is to enhance the desirability of pork and this will require a different approach than has been used to improve the quality of pork, and apart from reemphasising the importance of price in determining profitability, I will not address the matter any further in this paper. I have concentrated on what we have learned and achieved in terms of research and development and the relative impacts of the outcomes on the efficiency of pork production. Indeed, because of the likelihood that the global pork industry will be faced with higher feed costs and potentially the use of higher fibre ingredients in the foreseeable future I have tended to concentrate on factors likely to impact feed efficiency since improvement in this trait will likely deliver the greatest economic returns.

2. Effects of technology on the efficiency of the pork industry

Changes in live weight and whole herd feed conversion ratio for small to medium producers in the USA between 1985 and 2007 are shown in Table 1. Concommitant changes in the price of corn, cost of production, pig price and profit are also given in Table 1. There have been continual improvements in the

Table 1. Changes in pig performance, costs and profitability in the USA pork industry over 22 years (United Feeds producer records).

Year	Live weight	HFC[a]	Pig price (c/KG)	Corn ($/bushel)	COP (c/KG)[b]	Profit (c/KG)
1985	230	3.90	20.45	2.30	18.18	2.26
1986	230	3.80	22.67	2.30	17.64	5.98
1987	232	3.73	23.49	1.54	5.55	7.93
1988	236	3.69	19.50	2.28	18.05	1.47
1989	237	3.71	19.23	2.53	18.68	0.54
1990	239	3.73	24.17	2.46	17.96	6.21
1991	239	3.73	22.45	2.37	17.55	4.89
1992	241	3.62	18.86	2.41	17.19	1.66
1993	239	3.67	20.72	2.17	17.14	3.58
1994	245	3.66	18.77	2.49	18.18	0.58
1995	246	3.57	18.55	2.48	17.64	0.89
1996	247	3.57	23.99	3.89	22.27	1.47
1997	247	3.54	24.90	2.71	20.59	4.31
1998	251	3.47	16.87	2.33	18.05	-1.15
1999	253	3.48	14.33	1.96	16.10	-0.80
2000	253	3.41	19.68	1.88	16.01	3.63
2001	252	3.40	20.72	1.92	16.82	3.90
2002	253	3.40	15.87	2.18	17.69	-1.83
2003	260	3.32	18.00	2.35	17.73	0.23
2004	257	3.31	23.49	2.44	19.00	4.49
2005	259	3.29	23.04	2.03	16.87	2.13
2006	261	3.30	21.45	2.34	17.87	3.62
2007	?	?	?	4.13	?	?

[a] HFC: Herd Feed Conversion.
[b] COP: Cost of Production.

efficiency of production based on live weight and herd feed conversion which have increased and decreased by 14 kg (31 lb) and by 0.57 units respectively over the time period. These changes reflect technological advances and research and development outcomes over some 20 years and on average show that throughput has increased by at least 13% and feed efficiency by some 12%. It's interesting however, that there is no obvious relationship between these quite impressive improvements in production efficiency and profit which is most closely related to pig price and was highest in 1987. This apparent disconnect between profit and productive efficiency is because the impact of technological advances on profit are rather short lived and eventually change the structure of the industry, and their effects on supply tend to reduce price. In contrast, technical advances generated by research and development can markedly improve the national and global competitiveness of an industry and of individual businesses within an industry, and in particular, those who adopt new technology the quickest. For example, the top 10% of producers involved in the records summarised in Table 1 had a herd feed efficiency 15% lower and a profit 12.6% higher than the average of all participants for 2006.

In general, research and development and the evolution of feeding and management systems are driven by the major constraints facing an industry and would be expected to, and do, differ between countries such as Europe and the USA where historical feed costs have differed markedly as have legislative issues relating to welfare and the factors such as the use of antibiotics. Market factors and demands also differ between countries and such differences can make technologies developed in and for one country/market a lot less valuable in another. Nevertheless, apart from price and feed costs there are a number of key performance indicators (KPI) that affect profitability of any pork business and these are whole herd feed efficiency (HFC) and volume (pigs sold/sow/year and carcass weight). The volume component of the profit equation affects revenue, HFC and overhead costs and as such tends to have similar value globally. Based on the latest benchmarking results from Europe and North America, the Danish pork industry tends to have an advantage in terms of volume over The Netherlands, Canada and the USA. This is associated with excellent reproduction (pigs sold/sow/year) and a relatively heavy carcass weight. In contrast, because of relatively poor reproduction and light carcass weights the Australian pork industry trials Denmark by at least 25% in this KPI and as such reproduction is a high research priority. The KPI's for some selected countries for 2005 are given in Table 2.

Table 2. Key performance indicators and some cost information for 2005 for Ireland, Denmark, and the UK (British Pig Executive 2006) the USA (Agrimetrics 2005) and Australia (Australian Pork Limited – Pork Annual 2005).

KPI	Ireland	Denmark	UK	USA	Australia
Feed cost ($/tonne)[a]	292	237	252	155	235
HFC	3.72	4.03	4.31	4.2	4.2
Pigs sold/sow/yr	19.7	24.3	19.4	21	20.5
Carcass weight (kg)	76.6	80.2	76.2	92	72
Carcass/sow/y (kg)	1645	2058	1441	1932	1500
Cost of production ($/kg carcass weight)[a]	1.79	1.75	1.99	1.15	1.85
DE per kg carcass weight	49.6	56.2	56.3	61.0	56.7

[a] USA dollars.

The results suggest Ireland has a considerable advantage in terms of feed efficiency over the other countries included in the table. When the effect of dietary energy content is removed (Table 2) the results suggest the average amount of digestible energy (DE) used per kg of carcass weight produced was 49.6 MJ for Ireland which was some 12% lower that the next best (Denmark). This is impressive and may reflect the fact that Ireland has the highest feed costs though it is not possible to determine the reasons for the differences in efficiency.

It should be possible to reduce carcass DE efficiency to as low as 38 MJ/kg and researchers, geneticists and others involved in the technical and managerial sides of pork production should set similar targets and then investigate technologies and systems which allow them to be achieved cost effectively. Achieving such targets will require animals which are inherently efficient, technologies and systems which maximise animal health and minimise feed wastage and heat losses from the pig. Improving and/or maximising gut efficiency will play a role in achieving much better energy and feed efficiency than is currently the case, as will maximising the energy and nutrients extracted from grains and other feed ingredients.

The efficiency with which feed is used and HFC are clearly of major importance in countries where feed costs are high such as Australia, the UK and most of Europe. In the USA, less emphasis has been placed on feed efficiency particularly in genetic selection programmes largely because corn and feed costs have been traditionally low and more emphasis has been placed on growth rate and carcass lean content. Whilst the latter can never be ignored because it affects price, the effects of ethanol production in the USA has essentially doubled the price of corn in 2007 and corn prices are predicted to remain at 175% of traditional levels for the next five years. The impact of ethanol production on the amount of corn available for export from the USA will also affect grain prices globally during the same time period. It is changes of this magnitude which bring about major realignments in research priorities and there will be a far greater emphasis placed on improving feed conversion efficiency and the efficient use of 'by products' such as Distillers Dried Grains and Solubles (DDGS) and other materials in the North American industries. The latter might and probably should extend to the development of 'better' grains for pigs and a better understanding of how the different components of grains and by products might be used to enhance digestive efficiency and possibly even health. Personally I can't see any reason as to why the digestibility of grains and other dietary ingredients can't be markedly improved and systems and animals developed which markedly reduce the amount of energy required to produce a kg of carcass weight. Long term this is where the answers to further and more rapid improvements in the efficiency of pork production lie and highlights the timeliness and relevance of this seminar.

3. Factors affecting productivity

It has been my experience that the factors affecting the efficiency of pork production have changed little over time and in order of priority they are:
1. genetics/performance capabilities;
2. mortality/health;
3. management;
4. housing/environment;
5. reproduction;
6. nutrition.

The factors clearly interact with one another to affect the final outcome in terms of the KPI's discussed previously and we have a massive amount of information and research data on each of these factors. Furthermore it is likely that considerable improvement could be made if this information was applied correctly at the production level. In this respect the use of simulation models such as Auspig (Black *et al.*, 1986) and others developed in Europe integrate all the factors mentioned above to predict both biological and economic outcomes. Unfortunately, simulation models are underutilised in the pork industry and considerable potential exists for better application of current knowledge if the use of these models could be encouraged.

Factors such as the gut environment and how it might be modified to enhance health and/or performance is a relatively new area of research and its commercial implications remain to be fully understood or adopted to any extent. To date, most improvements in the performance and the efficiency of growing animals have been achieved by manipulating how absorbed nutrients are partitioned between protein, fat and maintenance. The best examples being the differences in feed efficiency and lean content exhibited by different sexes offered the same energy intake (Campbell *et al.*, 1985) and/or between different genotypes (Campbell and Taverner, 1986). Similarly, research with exogenous growth hormone administration has shown that at the same level of energy intake feed efficiency can be improved by 20-30% which is due almost entirely to the effects of growth hormone on protein deposition (Campbell *et al.*, 1989). The extent that technologies such as exogenous growth hormone might become commercially acceptable remains questionable, but the knowledge gained from earlier research in the area demonstrates the basic mechanisms underlying protein and energy metabolism and offers challenges and bench marks for Animal Scientists to aspire to. How endogenous growth hormone levels might be increased using nutritional and other technologies warrants further research.

Another relatively new area of research relates to the effects that differences between and within grains can have on performance. This is another area with particular relevance to the current seminar series and is discussed in more detail under a separate heading.

4. Looking back to go forward

4.1. Genetics and gender

The effect genetics can have on feed efficiency and growth is illustrated in Table 3 which shows the growth performance of gilts from two genetic lines between 20 and 110 kg live weight. The differences in feed: gain is quite marked and demonstrates the importance of genetics in determining the efficiency of commercial pork production. For example, the difference in feed: gain between

Table 3. Effects of genotype on the performance of gilts between 20 and 110 kg live weight (Campbell, unpublished results).

Performance traits	Genotype 1	Genotype 2
Growth rate (g/d)	820	927
Feed intake (kg/d)	2.19	2.08
Feed: gain	2.65	2.25
DE/kg gain	38.7	32.8

the two lines represents a difference in feed usage between 20 and 110 kg live weight of some 42 kg per pig or a 15% feed saving. The more efficient line also grew faster than the less efficient line. There have been some marked improvements in the performance capabilities of genetics available in the USA over the last seven years, and genetic improvement particularly in feed efficiency will play an increasingly important role in ensuring pork production is able to remain competitive against other meats in the higher cost grain environment we are all likely to face over the next 5-7 years. At the producer level, choosing the 'right' genetics could be a major factor determining longer term profitability and survival in the new industry.

Genetic improvement in feed efficiency essentially mimics the effects of exogenous growth hormone administration but enables improvements in virtually all aspects of production to be achieved at no additional cost to the producer and in a more acceptable way. The importance of genetics, and in particular, the role genetics will play in improving the efficiency with which energy is used by pork production should not be underestimated. It is likely that we will see changes in selection indexes towards feed efficiency and increased investment in the search for genetic markers for the same trait in the immediate and near future.

Similar differences in efficiency and in carcass lean content exist between the sexes and particularly between intact and castrated males. The latter is illustrated in Table 4 which shows published differences in feed efficiency and P2 backfat thickness between intact and castrated male pigs. Although the use of intact males for pork production has market and behavioural implications, surgical castration increases feed usage by 10-12% and reduces lean meat production by a similar amount. Consequently, the procedure should be questioned particularly under high feed cost situations. Surgical castration is also raising

Table 4. The reported advantages of intact males (boars) compared to surgical castrates for feed efficiency (% advantage of boars), P2 fat thickness and carcass fat content.

Live weight (kg)	Reference	Feed efficiency	P2	Carcass fat (%)
23-110	Turkstra *et al.* (2002)	+ 9.3%	zero	NR
29-105	Bonneau *et al.* (1994)	+ 11.4%	NR	-20.3%
53-100	Dunshea *et al.* (2001)	+ 12.2%	-23.6	NR
53-118	Dunshea *et al.* (2001)	+13.1%	-26.3	NR
77-108	Suster *et al.* (2006)	NR	-13.2	-21.5%

NR: not reported.

welfare concerns in parts of Europe and its is likely that in some countries surgical castration will not be permitted without anaesthesia and analgesia and may even be banned in the longer term. Whilst the latter has no implications with respect to the current seminar series the market and behavioural concerns surrounding the use of intact males for commercial production can be cost effectively overcome by immunocastration. The latter technology requires intact male pigs to be auto immunised against luteinising hormone releasing factor (LHRH) which inturn reduces testosterone and androsterone and skatole to levels equivalent to castrated males and as such enables the performance and lean advantages offered by intact males to be achieved without the potential taint and behavioural problems.

Whilst pigs have to be immunised twice with the second dose occurring 4-5 weeks before slaughter the technology is likely to receive more attention in counties currently surgically castrating male pigs as feed costs increase.

4.2. Nutrition and metabolism modification

4.2.1. Historical

There have been marked improvements in our understanding of the role nutrition plays in economically exploiting the genetic potential of pigs for growth and reproduction. Over the last 20 years the major advances in nutrition in chronological order have been:

1. The introduction of the ideal protein concept which simplified diet formulation and whilst the concept of an ideal amino acid balance has

little biological relevance at least to the pig, the concept has been adopted globally and has simplified diet formulation. Further research on amino acid balances however, is unlikely to further improve the cost effectiveness of diet formulation or animal performance.

2. The move from expressing dietary amino acid levels and requirements from total to available amino acids. The change markedly improved the accuracy of diet formulations and played a major role in supporting more consistent growth performance.
3. The discovery that, under amino acid sufficient situations, protein deposition in the pig is driven by energy intake and not protein or amino acid intake. The latter brought about the concept of amino acid: energy ratios in defining the growing pig's requirements and again simplified and improved the accuracy of diet formulation. The concept however, is often still misunderstood and this can result in nutritional strategies which lead to excess nitrogen output and often reduce, rather than improve, growth performance.
4. Establishment of the dietary amino acid and energy requirements of lactating gilts and the effects on subsequent reproductive performance (Tritton *et al.*, 1996). The original and subsequent research demonstrated a link between requirement and milk production and has been able to define the order of priority for amino acids under different levels of productivity.

These are all research outcomes that established the fundamental concepts of growth and development in pigs, dietary requirements and diet formulation. Whilst some continue to be investigated and refined, it is unlikely that major changes in the concepts will occur. In contrast, supporting research with metabolism modifiers such as growth hormone and ractopamine has provided us with a better understanding of the mechanisms underlying some of these concepts and the factors limiting further improvement in biological efficiency and performance. To a large extent the most limiting factor to further improvement in the efficiency of pork production remains the animal's inherent potential for protein deposition and any nutritional or other technology which enables this constraint to be removed or alleviated will likely be of significant economic value to pork production. For example, ractopamine which is used during the last 3-4 weeks of growth in many countries increases protein deposition and improves feed efficiency by 15 -25% and carcass weight by 4-6% and as such enables considerable improvements in production efficiency to be achieved. Specifically, the use of 5 ppm ractopamine in the last four weeks of commercial production has the potential to improve overall carcass feed efficiency by 4-5% while at the same time reducing overhead costs and increasing revenue. These are the types of improvements needed to help ensure pork production is able to keep pace with the changes in terms of trade likely to be experienced in the short to medium future.

The extent of the animal's inherent capacity for rapid, efficient growth or reproduction is limited by its environment and/or disease and is probably the area where the greatest improvements in pork production can be achieved at least in the shorter term. On the dietary side of the equation the likelihood of higher feed costs in the medium term suggests that the ability to extract more nutrients from ingredients and especially more fibrous ingredients and/or to use dietary components to enhance nutrient absorption will also contribute to more efficient and potentially profitable pork production.

4.2.2. Recent developments: dietary energy and commercial performance

Under ideal situations the growing pig generally responds to increasing dietary energy content by reducing its feed intake to maintain a relatively constant digestible energy (DE) intake (Campbell and Taverner, 1986). Consequently growth rate is largely unaffected by dietary DE. However, under group housing situations feed intake is generally lower and constrained by physical and behavioural factors, and recent evidence suggests that using diets of higher or high energy content particularly in the finishing phase of production can improve commercial performance. For example, Henman *et al.*, (1999) reported a linear response in the growth rate of group housed boars offered feed *ad libitum* to increase dietary DE content from 12.0 to 14.4 MJ/kg over a 42 day period commencing at 63 kg.

Over the same DE range, carcass weight increased from 74.3 to 80.5 kg and feed: gain declined from 3.08 to 2.65. The results have been confirmed in other studies (Campbell, 2005) and show that feed/energy intake which is the driver of protein deposition is constrained under commercial situations and a simple technology such as the use of higher energy diets has the potential firstly to more fully exploit the growth potential of modern genotypes and secondly to significantly increase the efficiency of commercial production.

The extent of the results reported by Henman *et al.*, (1999) were associated with energy *per se* and/or the effects of fat on metabolism and nutrient absorption remain to be established.

4.2.3. Recent developments: grains, enzymes and NIRS

One of the more intriguing research areas in the last 7-8 years has been the role grain and grains play in contributing to the variation in pig performance. For example, Cadogan *et al.* (1999) reported differences in the feed intakes of pigs offered diets based on 10 different wheat cultivars of 89%. The corresponding maximum difference in growth rate was 91%. In contrast, feed: gain was similar across the 10 grains and dry matter digestibility varied significantly but only marginally. The results were the first to highlight the extent grain type could have on the growth performance of pigs and led to the development of large research and development projects in Australia to establish the effects grains have on the performance of pigs, ruminants and poultry. The results to date have shown that grains most suitable for one species are not necessarily the most suitable for another, and that within grain DE content can vary by as much as 2.5 MJ/kg and feed intake by 30-40%.

The findings have important commercial and scientific implications. Firstly they suggest that using published DE values for grains in diet formulations will rarely result in the most cost effective outcome in terms of feed costs and will result in 'unexpected' variation in feed efficiency. Feed intake differences within and between grains will also contribute to variation in growth performance at the production level. The effects of enzyme supplementation will also vary depending on the intake characteristics of the grain and this has been shown by Choct *et al.* (1999) who reported that the use of a xylanase enzyme in diets based on low intake wheat markedly improved feed intake and growth rate. In contrast, the same enzyme was ineffective in improving the feed intake or growth of pigs offered diets based on higher intake wheats (Table 5). The results show both the variation in the feed intake differences between wheats in this case and the effect of the latter on the efficacy of exogenous enzyme supplementation.

The Pork CRC (Cooperative Research Centre) is investing in a number of related projects to develop near infrared spectroscopy (NIRS) calibrations to predict the DE and feed intake characteristics of grains for pigs.

The ability to rapidly determine these two characteristics of grains has the potential to revolutionise the cost effectiveness of diet formulation and to support more consistent and predictable pig performance. Grains with wide differences in DE and/or intake also provide excellent models for discovering the factors/chemical components of the grains contributing to the differences

Table 5. Effects of enzyme supplementation and wheat cultivar on the performance of male weaner pigs (Choct et al.*, 1999).*

Wheat	Enzyme	Daily gain (g)	Feed intake (g/d)	Feed : gain
Currawong	-	230 [a]	318 [a]	1.38
Currawong	+	466 [b]	516 [b]	1.23
Cocamba	-	425 [b]	540 [b]	1.27
Cocamba	+	445 [b]	521 [b]	1.20
Lawson	-	460 [b]	525 [b]	1.14
Lawson	+	479 [b]	570 [b]	1.20
Statistics				
Wheat (W)		***	***	NS
Enzyme (E)		***	***	NS
W XE		***	***	NS

[a-b]Means in the same column followed by different letters are significantly different.
*** (P <0.001); NS: not significant (P>0.05).

which may subsequently be included in grain breeding programmes and/or used to modify pig performance. There would also seem to be considerable potential for developing grains specific for pigs. These would have high DE content and high DE yield/hectare.

5. The future

The future needs of the global pork industry will vary depending on the major constraints facing each country and there will be intense competition for the export market(s). A common factor will remain the need for further improvements if feed efficiency and better feed/ingredient utilisation. At the animal level, technologies which enhance protein deposition capacity will improve feed efficiency. Additionally, at the environment level technologies/techniques which alleviate or remove external constraints on feed intake will have a greater effect on growth rate than feed efficiency, the value of which will vary more between countries than that of feed efficiency. The exception to the latter is disease which tends to have an adverse effect on the feed efficiency of the individual animal and an additional effect on commercial feed efficiency if the disease causes mortality. It is not within the scope of this paper or my expertise to discuss the heath status of the global pork industry. However, respiratory diseases appear to becoming increasingly more common and varied, and tend to be having a significant adverse effect on the productivity of pork production in a number of European countries and the USA.

5.1. The gut environment and improving gut efficiency

5.1.1. Enteric disease

The extent that nutritional strategies and nutrients might be able to alleviate some of the enteric diseases affecting pork production remains equivocal, but this is an area that has received considerable research effort in Europe because of changes in legislation affecting the use of antibiotics and growth promotants. Most of the enteric diseases affecting pigs are old diseases but do vary across the globe. In Australia *E. coli* remains a problem in newly weaned pigs and a similar situation probably exists globally. The Australian herd is also affected by swine dysentery (*Brachyspira hyodysenteriae*) which is rare in the USA and probably more prevalent in parts of Europe and the UK. Ileitis (*Lawsonia intracellularis*) appears common globally. These diseases certainly have an adverse effect on gut efficiency and biological or nutritional technologies that can alleviate them will have a positive effect on feed efficiency and overall performance and productivity.

Apart from dietary supplements such as Zinc oxide at high levels and possibly organic acids there is little conclusive evidence that *E. coli* diarrhoea can be controlled by nutritional means. In contrast, Pluske *et al.* (1996) reported that diets low in both non starch polysaccharides (NSP) and resistant starch (RS) may afford protection against *Brachyspira hyodysenteriae*. The exact mechanism for such protection remains to be defined but may be associated with the lack of fermentable substrate available in the large intestine and/or the effects of the fermentable carbohydrate on the proliferation of other bacterial species needed for *Brachyspira hyodysenteriae* to result in clinical disease. Whilst the mechanisms remain to be established, the results do offer hope that gut efficiency might be able to be improved via the nutritional control of some enteric pathogens. An alternative approach might involve the development of more highly digestible grains for pigs which would reduce total grain usage (but not total DE usage) and reduce the amount of substrate available for bacterial proliferation in both the small and large intestines.

5.1.2. Non-starch polysaccharides

In a more recent publication by Hogberg and Lindberg (2006) it was reported that diets high in both NSP and insoluble NSP (iNSP) supported much higher growth rates and feed efficiency in young pigs compared to diets high in NSP and similar performance as diets low in NSP. Whilst the effects of NSP on performance was confounded with differences in the grains used in the different diets, the authors reported that the excellent performance exhibited by pigs on the high NSP, iNSP diet was achieved despite the diet having a much lower DE than the low NSP diets. For example, the results suggested that the efficiency with which DE was utilised was 29% higher than for the control and low NSP diets. The findings have important commercial implications and it is possible that the results were associated with the effects of high NSP/iNSP diet on the gut environment since this diet promoted the production of lactic acid in the stomach and small intestine and butyric acid in the large intestine. The results suggest that with the correct combinations of NSP it may be possible to markedly improve the efficiency with which high fibre diets can be utilised in pig production. The changes in the gut environment reported by Hogberg and Lindberg (2006) also have implication with respect to the control of pathogenic bacteria possibly in pigs of all ages. The area clearly warrants further research.

We have also observed positive effects of higher Non digestible fibre (NDF) levels in diets for both weaner and grower pigs on feed efficiency and growth rate despite the calculated dietary DE content declining with increasing dietary NDF level (Campbell, unpublished results) suggesting that there are levels and types of fibre that either improve the utilisation of absorbed energy possibly though changes in the gut environment and animal health or by altering the rate of passage of digesta so that more nutrients are absorbed from the diet. In a recently reported study Spencer *et al.* (2007) similarly reported a linear improvement in the feed efficiency of weaner pigs in response to increasing dietary NDF in the form of distillers dried grains with solubles (DDGS) up to inclusion levels of 15% of the diet. The same authors also reported that including 30% DDGS in the diet offered to pigs in the first three weeks after weaning improved feed efficiency by 8.6%. These and the results of Hogberg and Lindberg (2006) certainly suggest that the effects of fibre level and type on nutrient absorption and utilisation are not fully understood. Considerable potential might exist for cost effectively improving feed efficiency without necessarily using diets of high DE content.

5.1.3. Exogenous enzymes

We are likely to see more interest in the use of exogenous enzymes especially in North America where DDGS (the by product of ethanol production) will receive increasing attention and be used at higher levels in pig diets. There is ample evidence that corn DDGS can replace up to 30% corn in diets for growing-finishing pigs with minimal effects on growth rate or live weight feed efficiency. However, because of its relatively high fibre content, DDGS levels above 20% of the diet generally have an adverse effect on dressing percentage and carcass weight (Linncan *et al.*, 2007). Recent publications suggest that including cellulase/xylanase enzymes in the diets offered to finisher and weaner pigs can alleviate the adverse effects of higher DDGS levels on carcass yield (Gaines *et al.*, 2007) and improve the growth rate of younger pigs (Spencer *et al.*, 2007).

It was mentioned previously that variability in the performance supporting characteristics within and between grains is a major factor affecting the responsiveness of pigs to exogenous dietary enzyme supplementation (Choct *et al.*, 1999). Having the ability to rapidly determine the likelihood of the responsiveness of a grain (ingredient) to enzyme supplementation will allow this old technology to be better exploited.

6. Conclusions

Based on previous experience in research and development and in commercial pork production, the major factor which has resulted in the greatest improvements in animal performance has been enhancing protein deposition capacity largely through genetics. However, some countries have decided to take advantage of the higher protein deposition capacity of intact males by ceasing surgical castration. Others have adopted technologies such as exogenous growth hormone administration and ractopamine use. In the longer term, genetics will continue to improve and technologies whether nutritional or otherwise, which enhance protein deposition will have a positive effect on feed efficiency and overall productivity.

Removing commercial constraints preventing full expression of the pigs inherent protein deposition capacity will also improve the efficiency of pork production. Physical and behavioural constraints on feed intake can be alleviated through rather simple nutritional strategies such as the use of higher energy diets especially for heavier pigs.

Disease is probably the biggest potential constraint on the overall efficiency of pork production. The control of respiratory diseases will rely on the development of appropriate vaccines whilst there is some evidence that some of the enteric diseases may be 'controlled' by nutritional means. Further research is required to better understand the mechanisms involved in the pathogenesis of the common enteric disease organisms and how/where nutrition/nutrients may have a role in alleviating this constraint to gut efficiency.

There is increasing evidence that the characteristics of grains can affect both feed intake and feed efficiency and considerable potential would seem to exist for improving the consistency and efficiency of pork production by better understanding the components of grains which result in the wide variation in both energy availability and feed intake. Indeed, such information will enhance the efficiency and cost effectiveness of exogenous enzyme supplementation and potentially throw light on the role of different grain components on gut efficiency.

It has always been my belief that if economically possible dietary fibre should be kept as low as possible in the diets for all classes of growing pigs since all the old evidence suggests that increasing dietary fibre reduces growth performance, increases feed usage and the associated milling and delivery costs and most importantly reduces carcass weight. However, it is likely that grain costs will increase interest in and the use of, more fibrous ingredients in the foreseeable future so we need to think about how such ingredients can be used more efficiently. Some of the recent research on NSP and the nature of NSP suggest there may be previously unrealised potential to improve the gut environment and the utilisation of absorbed energy possibly through improved 'health'. There is also evidence that different fibre components can be used to improve gut efficiency by manipulating the rate of digesta through the digestive tract. These are exciting prospects but require further research.

Overall, some things affecting the efficiency of pork production never change and it is generally at our expense when we ignore these. However, changes in the market place change the order of priority for such technologies/factors and how they might be employed. Enhancing gut efficiency is a relatively new area of research but the results discussed on the role of grains and fibre on feed intake and energetic efficiency suggest this is an area which could play a major role in improving the efficiency of pork production in the future.

References

Black, J.L., Campbell, R.G., Williams, I.H., James, K.J. and Davies, G.T. (1986). Simulation of energy and amino acid utilisation in the pig. *Research and Development in Agriculture* **3:** 121-145.

Bonneau, M., Dufour, R., Chouvet, C., Roulet, C., Meadus, W. and Squires, E. (1994). The effects of immunization against luteinizing hormone-releasing hormone on performance, sexual development, and levels of boar taint-related compounds in intact male pigs. *Journal of Animal Science* **72:** 14-20.

Cadogan, D.J., Choct, M., Campbell, R.G. and Kershaw, S. (1999). Effects of new season's wheat on the growth performance of young male pigs. In: *Manipulating Pig Production VII* (ed. P.D. Cranwell), Australasian Pig Science Association: Werribee, Vic. Australia. pp. 40.

Campbell, R.G. (2005). Fats in pig diets: beyond their contribution to energy content. *Recent Advances in Animal Nutrition in Australia* **15:** 15-19.

Campbell, R.G., Taverner, M.R. and Curic, D.M. (1985). Effects of sex and energy intake between 45 and 90 kg live weight on protein deposition in growing pigs. *Animal Production* **40:** 497-454.

Campbell, R.G. and Taverner, M.R. (1986). The effects of dietary fibre, source of fat and dietary energy content of the voluntary energy intake and performance of growing pigs. *Animal Production* **42:** 327-337.

Campbell, R.G., Taverner, M.R. and Curic, D.M. (1984). Effects of sex and energy intake between 48 and 90 kg live weight on protein deposition, growth performance and body composition of growing pigs. *Animal production* **38:** 211-220.

Campbell, R.G. Steele, N.C., Caperna, T.J., Mc Murtry, J.P., Solomon, M.B. and Mitchell, A.D. (1988). Interrelationships between energy intake and exogenous porcine growth hormone administration on the performance body composition and protein and energy metabolism of growing pigs weighting 25 to 55 kg. *Journal of Animal Science* **66:** 1643-1651.

Campbell, R.G., Steele, N.C., Caperna, T.J. Mc Murtry, J.P Solomon, M.B. and Mitchell, A.D. (1989). Interrelationships between sex and exogenous porcine growth hormone administration on the performance body composition and protein and fat accretion of growing pigs. *Journal of Animal Science* **67:** 177-186.

Choct, M., Cadogan, D.J., Campbell, R.G. and Kershaw, S. (1999). Enzymes can eliminate the difference in the nutritive value of wheat for pigs. In: *Manipulating Pig Production VII* (ed. P.D. Cranwell). Australasian Pig Science Association: Werribee, Vic. Australia. pp. 40.

Dunshea F.R., Colantoni, C., Howard, K., McCauley, I., Jackson P., Long K.A., Lopaticki, S., Nugent, E.A., Simons, J.A., Walker, J. and Hennessy D.P. (2001). Vaccination of boars with a GnRH vaccine (Improvac) eliminates boar taint and increases growth performance. *Journal of Animal Science* **79:** 2524-2535.

Gaines, A.M., Petersen, G.I., Spencer, J.D. and Augspurger, N.R. (2007). Use of corn distillers dried grains with solubles (DDGS) in finishing pigs. *Journal of Animal Science, Abstracts* **85:** 55.

Henman, D.J., Argent, C.J. and Bryden, W.L. (1999). Response of male and female finisher pigs to dietary energy density. In: *Manipulating Pig Production VII* (ed. P.D. Cranwell). Australasian Pig Science Association: Werribee, Vic. Australia. pp. 40.

Hogberg A. and Lindberg J.E. (2006). The effect of level and type of cereal non-starch polysaccharides on the performance, nutrient utilization and gut environment of pigs around weaning. *Animal feed Science and Technology* **127:** 200-219.

Linneen, S.K., Tokach, M.D., DeRouchey. J.M., Dritz, S.S., Goodband, R.D., Nelssen, J.L. and Main, R.G. (2007). Effects of dried distillers grain with solubles on grow-finish performance. *Journal of Animal Science, Abstracts* **85:** 54.

Pluske, J.R., Siba, P.M., Pethick, D.W., Durmic, Z., Mullan, B.P. and Hampson, D.J. (1996). The incidence of swine dysentery in pigs can be reduced by feeding diets that limit the amount of fermentable substrate entering the large intestine. *Journal of Nutrition* **126:** 2920-2933.

Spencer, J.D., Petersen, G.I., Gaines, A.M. and Augspurger, N.R. (2007). Evaluation of different strategies for supplementing distiller's dried grains with solubles to nursery pig diets. *Journal of Animal Science, Abstracts* **85:** 55.

Suster, D., Leury, B.J., Kerton, D.J., Borg, M.R., Butler, K.L. and Dunshea, F.R. (2006). Longitudinal DXA measurements demonstrate lifetime differences in lean and fat tissue deposition in individually penned and group-penned boars and barrows. *Australian Journal of Agricultural Research* **57:** 1009-1015.

Tritton, S.M., King, R.H., Campbell, R.G., Edwards, A.C. and Hughes, P.E. (1996). The effects of dietary protein and energy levels of diets offered during lactation on the lactation and subsequent reproductive performance of first-litter sows. *Journal of Animal Science* **62:** 573-579.

Turkstra, J.A., Zeng, X.Y, Van Diepen, J.Th.M., Jongbloed, A.W., Oonk, H.B., Van de Wiel, D.F.M. and Meloen, R.H. (2002). Performance of male pigs immunized against GnRH is related to the time of onset of biological response. *Journal of Animal Science* **80:** 2953-2959.

Host and intestinal microbiota negotiations in the context of animal growth efficiency

H. Rex Gaskins
Departments of Animal Sciences and Pathobiology, Division of Nutritional Sciences, Institute for Genomic Biology, University of Illinois at Urbana-Champaign, 1207 West Gregory Drive, Urbana, Illinois 61801, USA

1. Introduction

The complex relationship between the animal host and the non-pathogenic, indigenous (autochthonous) microbiota[1] residing in its gastrointestinal (GI) tract presents an intriguing immunological paradox. Despite being exquisitely capable of distinguishing self from nonself, the host tolerates the residence of an antigenically variable and metabolically complex microbiota. The resident microbiota is advantaged by a rich and continuous supply of nutrients as well as a favourable environment in which to live. In turn, the resident microbiota contributes to the nutritional economy of the host and plays a critical role in host resistance to enteric pathogens (Bealmear, 1981; Berg, 1996; Bry *et al.*, 1996; Bryant, 1974; Cebra, 1999; Cebra *et al.*, 1980, Savage, 1986). That such a mutualistic relationship exists implies that the protective and nutritional benefits of the microbiota are greater than the pathogenic threat offered by these foreign organisms. Indeed, all animals have, and seemingly require, a long-term cooperative association with indigenous microbes in the GI tract.

Studies with gnotobiotic[2] animal models demonstrate most conclusively that indigenous microbes stimulate the normal maturation of host tissues and provide key defense and nutritional functions (Beaver and Wostmann, 1962; Gordon *et al.*, 1966; Pabst *et al.*, 1988; Rothkotter and Pabst, 1989; Rothkotter *et al.*, 1991; Wostmann and Bruckner-Kardoss, 1959; Thorbecke, 1959). This mutualistic relationship has been selected over evolutionary time resulting in a stable microbiota in mature individuals that is generally similar in composition and function in a diverse range of animal species (Zoetendal *et al.*, 2004). Despite evolutionary stability, the intestinal microbiota develops in individual animals

[1] The suggestion of Lee (1984) that *microbiota* is the taxonomically correct term to describe the complex intestinal microbial community is followed.

[2] Harboring a defined and specific microbiota comprised of one or more organisms.

in a characteristic successional pattern that requires substantial adaptation by the host during early life. The impact of the developing microbiota as well as the metabolic activities of climax communities require special consideration when viewed in the context of animal production in which efficiency of growth is a primary objective (Gaskins, 2001).

Carriage of microbial populations capable of utilising refractory plant components enabled feral pigs to exploit distinct habitats thereby enhancing survival and reproductive success. Animal growth efficiency is, however, a concept introduced only upon domestication of animals as a food animal. These issues provoke consideration of an optimal gut microbiota for intestinal health versus its effects on the efficiency of gastrointestinal and whole body growth throughout the productive life cycle of a pig. However, the normal microbiota of the pig intestine has received surprisingly little attention from an animal growth perspective.

2. The gut microbiota is competitive with the host in the small intestine but cooperative in the large intestine

Much of our knowledge of host-microbe interactions in the intestine is based on *in vitro* culture-based studies. These techniques are subject to several biases, but until recently were the microbiologist's major tool. Culture-based studies have shown that microbial activity in the small intestine tends to be competitive with the host for energy and amino acids (Hedde and Lindsey, 1986). For example, bacterial utilisation of glucose to produce lactic acid reduces the energy available to the host animal (Saunders and Sillery, 1982). Lactic acid also enhances peristalsis, thus increasing the rate of nutrient transit in the gut (Saunders and Sillery, 1982). As much as 6% of the net energy in pig diets can be lost due to bacterial utilisation of glucose in the small intestine (Vervaeke *et al.*, 1979). Amino acids, which are also degraded by small intestinal bacteria, are made unavailable to the pig and produce toxic metabolites such as ammonia, cadaverine, and *p*-cresol. Although microbial activity in the caecum and colon tends to be cooperative with the host (Hedde and Lindsay, 1986), with estimates up to 5-20% of the pig's total energy being provided by fermentation by distal gut bacteria (Friend *et al.*, 1963), the small intestine is the principal site of nutrient and energy absorption. Further, bacterial populations in the small intestine are several orders of magnitude less dense than in the large intestine (Stewart, 1996). Thus, the benefits of growth-promoting antibiotics may result from a substantial decrease in bacterial populations and consequent alterations in epithelial functions in the small intestine, while changes in large intestine microbial populations exert less impact on whole animal growth. In support of this hypothesis, most of the growth-promoting antibiotics target Gram-positive organisms, and the small intestinal microbiota consists predominantly of Gram-positive bacteria (Stewart, 1996.) Again, available data on the spatial distribution of bacterial groups along the GI tract were generated via culture-based techniques and are thus undoubtedly biased. Continued use of molecular-based techniques will enable a more accurate evaluation of the concept that animal growth may be influenced by the spatial density and perhaps taxonomic composition of the microbiota along the GI tract.

3. Gut bacteria and intestinal inflammation

Intestinal bacteria play an important role in the development of the intestinal immune system (Gaskins, 1997). This immunogenic role of the gut microbiota is most clearly observed in the immaturity of the gut immune system in Germ-free (GF) animals, which have underdeveloped intestinal lymphoid tissues, substantially decreased numbers of lymphocytes (B and T-cells), and low antibody concentrations (Wostmann, 1996). These immune parameters convert to the normal state when GF animals are associated with a full complement of intestinal bacteria (Carter and Pollard, 1971). Studies in which individual species or known groups of bacteria have been introduced into GF animals have shown that different bacterial species may be very immunogenic, moderately immunogenic, or weakly/nonimmunogenic (McCracken and Gaskins, 1999). Obviously, bacterial stimulation of mucosal immune system development is crucial for protective immunity. However, one potential mechanism by which growth-promoting antibiotics may exert their effects is to decrease immunogenic bacteria inhabiting the small intestine. By limiting growth of small intestinal bacteria, growth-promoting antibiotics may decrease the energetic costs associated with the constitutive, low-level inflammation in the gut of conventional animals. Thus, the trade-off between the costs of local inflammation versus the necessity of immune competence becomes an issue which will be influenced by the housing environment. Stahly and co-workers (1995) studied the impact of tylosin on rate, efficiency, and composition of growth in pigs subject to either a conventional or medicated early-weaning protocol. They determined that feeding tylosin improved weight gain and feed efficiency, increased body protein, and reduced body fat in both groups, but the magnitude of response was highest for the conventionally-weaned and perhaps more immunologically-challenged group. Roura and co-workers

(1992) studied the relationship of the state of immune activation in broiler chickens to the growth-permitting ability of antibiotics. They also present data consistent with the hypothesis that feeding antibiotics may permit growth by preventing immunogenic stress and associated metabolic changes brought about by cytokines.

4. Bacteria alter intestinal epithelial turnover and maintenance energy requirements

The epithelial lining of the GI tract is characterised by a high cell turnover rate and the constant production of a protective mucus coat. Together these two physiological processes provide effective innate defence against luminal threats including those emanating from normal gut bacteria. In fact, epithelial cell turnover and secretory activity are both profoundly affected by the numbers, types, and spatial distribution of GI bacteria, with the latter microbial features being influenced by both exogenous and endogenous (host-derived) nutrients. Innate defence functions afforded by the epithelium are provided at the expense of animal growth efficiency. Specifically, GI tissues represent only 5% of body weight (approximate) but they receive a disproportionate fraction of cardiac output and contribute 15-35% of whole body oxygen consumption and protein turnover (Ebner *et al.*, 1994; Edelstone and Holzman, 1981; McNurlan and Garlick, 1980). Only 10% of the total protein synthesised by the GI tract is accumulated as new mass (Reeds *et al.*, 1993); most proteins are lost in sloughed epithelial cells or as secreted products such as mucus.

The presence of normal gut bacteria contributes to a thicker gut wall, heavier intestinal weight, reduced absorptive capacity, and a more rapid mucosal cell replacement rate (Commission on Antimicrobial Feed Additives, 1997). Mechanisms underlying these effects are generally unknown but may result from host responses to bacterial antigens or their metabolic end products as discussed above. Based on data from GF animals, it has been assumed that feeding antibiotics can reduce or prevent these negative effects. The most obvious difference between GF and conventional animals is a thinner wall of the small intestine, with a reduction in connective tissue and lymphoid elements (reviewed by Coates, 1980). Microscopic evaluation of GF intestine reveals a more regular and slender villus structure, with a thinner lamina propria. Further, the rate of renewal of epithelial cells is slower in GF animals, which may have a beneficial effect on basal energy expenditure and energetic efficiency of nutrient utilisation. These observations are consistent with the view of Reeds and coworkers (1993) that in rapidly growing young animals, the GI tract and the skeletal musculature draw from the same limited supply of nutrients and are, in effect, competitors for the deposition of nutrients.

Specific-pathogen-free (SPF) pigs have been shown to have lower maintenance energy requirements than normally-reared littermates (Verstegen *et al.*, 1981). Piglets used in the study were delivered by hysterectomy. Half of each litter was transferred to a foster sow on a commercial pig farm (Group 1) and the other half was maintained under SPF conditions (Group 2) presumably resulting in early differences in gut microbial populations. At 10-12 weeks of age, animals from each group were transferred to separate respiratory chambers and were raised to approximately 105 kg. The groups remained strictly isolated from each other and under strict hygienic conditions, with incoming air treated with UV light and feed irradiated. At 105 kg body weight, empty gut weight (2872 *vs.* 3003 g) and large intestine mesenteric lymph node weights (51 vs. 84 g) were both lower in SPF-reared animals than in conventional pigs (Verstegen *et al.*, 1981). Maintenance energy requirements were lower in the SPF group, consistent with the possibility that mutualistic gut microbes affect maintenance energy and may have a lasting effect even under strict hygienic conditions during the growing and finishing period.

5. Summary and outlook

The intestinal microbiota provides for its host important protective functions. Indigenous bacteria are capable of directly blocking enteric pathogens from colonising the intestine, and they are the primary stimuli for the development and maintenance of a local and multi-tiered defence system comprised of a full array of innate and acquired immunologic functions. The intestinal microbiota also contributes to host nutrition through the production of short chain fatty acids (SCFAs), vitamins, and amino acids. However, the cooperative or beneficial effects of the normal microbiota come at a cost to the host in terms of nutrient utilisation, epithelial and mucus turnover, detoxification of bacterial catabolites, and the continual production of resident inflammatory and immune cells. The costs of maintaining a balanced relationship or state of détente, between the host and its intestinal microbiota becomes a key consideration when maximising the efficiency of animal growth is a primary objective.

Numerous management practices likely directly or indirectly destabilise host-microbiota relationships, resulting in intestinal inflammation and possibly disruption of normal growth. Management practices having a direct influence on the microbiota include diet changes associated with life cycle feeding strategies and the inclusion of oral antibiotics in animal diets. Indeed, the growth-promoting effects of antibiotics are consistent with the possibility that the normal microbiota negatively impacts the energetics of animal growth. However, surprisingly little is known about the effects of sub-therapeutic levels of antibiotics on the normal gut microbiota. Management practices possibly having an indirect influence on microbial stability in the gut include those that disrupt normal feed and water intake patterns because of the stresses associated with herd rearrangement or relocation through the production life cycle. Often, herd rearrangement and diet changes are implemented concurrently and accompanied by overt intestinal inflammation.

These issues bring to mind the concept of an optimal microbiota for intestinal health versus the efficiency of gastrointestinal and whole body growth throughout the productive life cycle of a pig. However, many key questions require answers before the concept of an optimal gut microbiota for animal growth can be transferred to practical applications for the pig industry. For example, little is known about either bacterial cues or host response pathways that underlie host-microbe homeostasis. The microbial groups colonising the mucus layer and the epithelial surface remain undefined. There is very little information on animal-to-animal variation in microbiota profiles, particularly in relation to individual variation in growth efficiency among animals. The extent to which microbial populations remain stable within individual animals throughout the production life cycle is also mostly unknown. The influence of diet on microbial populations is poorly understood, particularly those habitats (e.g., small intestine) that may compete with the host for nutrients or otherwise decrease growth. The nutritional costs to the host of the microbiota at various developmental stages remain undefined, as does the energetic costs associated with intestinal inflammation in response to disruption of normal host-microbe relationships. The availability of molecular-based microbial ecology techniques provides exciting new options for addressing such questions. Answers should enable careful reconsideration of the role of the intestine as a growth-regulating organ. Novel strategies to enhance the efficiency of growth in livestock species may be identified in the process.

References

Bealmear, P.M. (1981). Host defense mechanisms in gnotobiotic animals. In: *Immunologic Defects in Laboratory Animals*, (Eds. M.E. Gershwin and B. Merchant). Plenum Press, New York. pp. 261–350.

Beaver M.H. and Wostmann B.S. (1962). Histamine and 5-hydroxytryptamine in the intestinal tract of germ-free animals, animals harbouring one microbial species and conventional animals. *British Journal of Pharmacology and Chemotherapy* **19:** 385-393.

Berg R.D. (1996). The indigenous gastrointestinal microflora. *Trends in Microbiology* **4:** 430-435.

Bry, L., Falk, P.G., Midtvedt, T. and Gordon, J.I. (1996). A model of host-microbial interactions in an open mammalian ecosystem. *Science* **273:** 1380-1383.

Bryant, M.P. (1974). Nutritional features and ecology of predominant anaerobic bacteria of the intestinal tract. *American Journal of Clinical Nutrition* **27:** 1313-1319.

Carter, P.B. and Pollard, M. (1971). Host responses to 'normal' microbial flora in germ-free mice. *Research Journal of the Reticuloendothelial Society* **9:** 580-587.

Cebra, J.J., Gearhart, P.J., Halsey, J.F., Hurwitz, J.L. and Shahin, R.D. (1980). Role of environmental antigens in the ontogeny of the secretory immune response. *Journal of the Reticuloendothelial Society* **28:** 61s-71s.

Cebra, J.J. (1999). Influences of microbiota on intestinal immune system development. *American Journal of Clinical Nutrition* **69:** 1046S-51S.

Coates, M.E. (1980). The gut microflora and growth. In: *Growth in Animals* (Ed. T.L.J. Lawrence) Butterworths, Boston, pp. 175-188.

Coates, M.E., Fuller, R., Harrison, G.F., Lev, M. and Suffolk, S.F. (1963). A comparison of the growth of chicks in the Gustafsson germ-free apparatus and in a conventional environment, with and without dietary supplements of penicillin. *British Journal of Nutrition* **17:** 141-151.

Commission on Antimicrobial Feed Additives. (1997). Antimicrobial Feed Additives. *Government Official Reports, SOU* 1997:132, Ministry of Agriculture, Stockholm.

Ebner, S., Schoknecht, P., Reeds, P. and Burrin, D. (1994). Growth and metabolism of gastrointestinal and skeletal muscle tissues in protein-malnourished neonatal pigs. *American Journal of Physiology* **266:** R1736-1743.

Edelstone, D.I. and Holzman, I.R. (1981). Oxygen consumption by the gastrointestinal tract and liver in conscious newborn lambs. *American Journal of Physiology* **240:** G297-304.

Friend, D.W., Cunningham, H.M. and Nicholson, J.W.G. (1963). The production of organic acids in the pig. *Canadian Journal of Animal Science* **43:** 156-168.

Gaskins, H.R. (1997). Immunological aspects of host/microbiota interactions at the intestinal epithelium. In: *Gastrointestinal Microbiology. (vol. 2). Gastrointestinal Microbes and Host Interactions* (Eds. R.I. Mackie, B.A. White and R.E. Isaacson). Chapman and Hall, New York. pp. 537-587.

Gaskins, H.R. (2001). Intestinal bacteria and their influence on swine growth. In: *Swine Nutrition.* (Eds. A.J. Lewis and L.L. Southern). CRC Press, Boca Raton, pp. 585-608.

Gordon, H.A., Bruckner-Kardoss, E., Staley, T.E., Wagner, M. and Wostmann, B.S. (1966). Characteristics of the germfree rat. *Acta Anatomica* **64:** 367-89.

Hedde, R.D. and Lindsey, T.O. (1986). Virginiamycin: A nutritional tool for swine production. *Agri-Practice* **7(3-4).**

Lee, A. (1984). Neglected niches: The microbial ecology of the gastrointestinal tract. In: *Advances in Microbial Ecology, Vol 8.* (Ed. K.C. Marshall). Plenum Press, New York, pp. 115-162.

McCracken, V.J. and Gaskins, H.R. (1999). Probiotics and the immune system. In: *Probiotics: A Critical Review.* (Ed. G.W. Tannock) Horizon Scientific Press, Norfolk, England, pp. 85-112.

McNurlan, M.A. and Garlick, P.J. (1980). Contribution of rat liver and gastrointestinal tract to whole-body protein synthesis in the rat. *Biochemical Journal* **186:** 381-383.

Pabst, R., Geist, M., Rothkotter, H.J. and Fritz, F.J. (1988). Postnatal development and lymphocyte production of jejunal and ileal Peyer's patches in normal and gnotobiotic pigs. *Immunology* **64:** 539-544.

Reeds, P.J., Burrin, D.G., Davis, T.A. and Fiorotto, M.L. (1993). Postnatal growth of gut and muscle: competitors or collaborators. *Proceedings of the Nutrition Society* **52:** 57-67.

Rothkotter, H.J. and Pabst, R. (1999). Lymphocyte subsets in jejunal and ileal Peyer's patches of normal and gnotobiotic minipigs. *Immunology* **67:** 103-108.

Rothkotter, H.J., Ulbrich, H. and Pabst, R. (1991). The postnatal development of gut lamina propria lymphocytes: Number, proliferation, and T and B cell subsets in conventional and germ-free pigs. *Pediatric Research* **29:** 237-242.

Roura, E., Homedes, J. and Klasing, K.C. (1992). Prevention of immunologic stress contributes to the growth-permitting ability of dietary antibiotics in chicks. *Journal of Nutrition* **122:** 2383-2390.

Saunders, D.R. and Sillery, J. (1982). Effect of lactate on structure and function of the rat intestine. *Digestive Diseases* **27:** 33-41.

Savage, D.C. (1986). Gastrointestinal microflora in mammalian nutrition. *Annual Review of Nutrition* **6:** 155-178.

Stahly, T.S., Williams, N.H. and Zimmermann, D.R. (1995). Impact of tylosin on rate, efficiency and composition of growth in pigs with a low or high level of immune system activation. *Journal of Animal Science* 73 **(Suppl. 1):** 84.

Stewart, C.S. (1996). Microorganisms in hindgut fermentors. In: *Gastrointestinal Microbiology. (vol. 2). Gastrointestinal Microbes and Host Interactions* (Eds. R.I. Mackie, B.A. White and R.E. Isaacson). Chapman and Hall, New York. pp. 142-186.

Thorbecke, G.J. (1959). Some histological and functional aspects of lymphoid tissue in germfree animals. I. morphological studies. *Annals of the New York Academy of Sciences* **78:** 237-246.

Verstegen, M.W.A., Van der Hel, W. and Brandsma, H.A. (1981). Energy balance traits in SPF (specific pathogen free) and normally reared littermates during the growing and finishing period. In: *Metabolic Disorders in Farm Animals.* (Eds. E. Gieseke, G. Dirksen, and M. Stangassinger). pp. 161-164.

Vervaeke, I.J., Decuypere, J.A., Dierick, N.A. and Henderickx, H.K. (1979). Quantitative *in vitro* evaluation of the energy metabolism influenced by virginiamycin and spiramycin used as growth promoters in pig nutrition. *Journal of Animal Science* **49:** 846-856.

Wostmann, B. and Bruckner-Kardoss, E. (1959). Development of cecal distention in germ-free baby rats. *American Journal of Physiology* **197:** 1345-1346.

Wostmann, B.S. (1996). Immunology, including radiobiology and transplantation. In: *Germfree and Gnotobiotic Animal Models.* (Ed. B.S. Wostmann) CRC Press, Boca Raton, FL., pp. 101-125.

Zoetendal, E.G., Collier, C.T., Koike, S., Mackie, R.I. and Gaskins, H.R. (2004). Molecularecological analysis of the gastrointestinal microbiota: a review. *Journal of Nutrition* **134:** 465-472.

Gut development: interactions between nutrition, gut health and immunity in young pigs

J.R. Pluske
School of Veterinary and Biomedical Sciences, Murdoch University, WA 6150, Australia

1. Introduction

The gastrointestinal tract (GIT) of the young pig is a complex interface between the animal and its environment, and is continuously challenged with a diverse array of dietary and microbial antigens. These antigens play a critical role in moulding both the structure and function, and in particular barrier function, of the intestine and its associated immune system. Major alterations in GIT biology occur concurrently with the abrupt dietary and environmental changes caused by birth and weaning, which are associated with heightened susceptibility to disease but importantly, are also recognised as critical periods during which immune defence mechanisms essential to the survival and performance of animals, are both primed and activated (Kelly and King, 2001). There is renewed appreciation, particularly in light of bans/restrictions on the use of antibiotic feed additives and heavy metals, that multi-disciplinary investigations to address the interactions between nutrition, the microbiota and immunity, particularly during early neonatal and post-natal life, are required to make advances in production and welfare.

In this light, it is crucial to acknowledge that commensal and pathogenic bacteria have evolved a diverse range of mechanisms that promote their survival within the ecosystem of the GIT (Kelly and Conway, 2005). Bacteria can produce a vast array of cytokine-inducing or cytokine-modulating molecules that will regulate or direct the host response. Some of these factors may promote the virulence and pathogenic potential of bacteria but others may facilitate the maintenance of the indigenous microflora by beneficially regulating the immunoinflammatory status of the GIT (Kelly and King, 2001). Indeed, there is a view that some enteric bacteria actually also help reduce maintenance costs of the gastrointestinal system (Kelly and King, 2001). Further discussion is beyond the scope of this paper and will be reviewed by Gaskins (2008) in another paper in these proceedings. The purpose of this paper is to briefly review GIT immunity and then explore some of the relationships between nutrition and GIT immune function in the young pig.

2. Defence mechanisms of the gastrointestinal tract

Numerous authors (e.g. Gaskins, 1998; Kelly and King, 2001; Dvorak *et al.*, 2006) have previously described the basic principles associated with defence mechanisms in the GIT of the young pig. To briefly summarise, the GIT is usually thought of primarily as an organ of digestion and absorption, but it is an extremely metabolically active organ and plays a very important 'barrier' role, protecting the body from harmful intra-luminal pathogens and large antigenic molecules (Gaskins, 1998). The external surface of the intestine comprises a single layer of epithelial cells that, along with the underlying lamina propria and muscularis mucosae, comprises the mucosa (mucous membrane; Mowat and Viney, 1997; Pluske *et al.*, 1997). The mucosal epithelium varies with location along the GIT and broadly reflects the functional requirements for digestion and absorption of nutrients and microbial defence. These two functions, i.e. as a nutrient absorber and microbial barrier, create a conflict in function that necessitates a complex system of physical, biochemical, and cellular mechanisms for protection of the intestinal mucosa from invading pathogens (Dvorak *et al.*, 2006).

The epithelium of the small intestine has evolved to be specialised for absorptive and secretory functions, from the duodenum to the ileum. The epithelium consists of a single layer of tall columnar cells arranged as villi projecting into the lumen and intestinal glands or crypts. The luminal border of the absorptive cells consists of microvilli, which greatly increase the absorptive area of the epithelium. Goblet cells secrete mucus, which protects the epithelium by binding to and slowing the mobility of pathogens. Lysozyme secreted by Paneth cells in the crypts and proline-rich peptide defensins such as PR-39 are antibacterial factors also present in the mucous layer (summarised in Dvorak *et al.*, 2006).

The gut mucosal barrier comprises an array of immunological and non-immunological protective components, the former being divided into local and systemic components and the latter comprising mechanical and chemical barriers, as well as intra-luminal bacteria (Rowlands and Gardiner, 1998; Table 1). The maintenance of normal epithelial cell structure prevents trans-epithelial migration of particles from the gut lumen, and the preservation of tight junctions between the cells prevents movement through the paracellular channels (Van

Table 1. Components of the gut mucosal barrier (from Rowlands and Gardiner, 1998).

Immunological	Non-immunological
Local	**Mechanical**
Gut-associated lymphoid tissue	Healthy enterocyte
Intra-epithelial lymphocytes	Tight junction
Submucosal aggregates	Cell turnover
Peyer's patches	Normal motility
Mesenteric lymph nodes	**Chemical**
Secretory IgA	Gastric acidity
Systemic	Salivary lysozyme
Circulatory lymphocytes	Lactoferrin
Hepatic Kupffer cells	Mucus secretion
	Bile salts
	Bacteriological
	Aerobic micro-organisms
	Anaerobic micro-organisms

IgA: immunoglobulin A.

Leeuwen *et al.*, 1994). Acid secretion in the stomach, alkali secretions in the small bowel and mucus production throughout the GIT provide additional protection (summarised in Gaskins, 1998).

2.1. Development of the GIT immune system

Pigs have evolved many immunological characteristics in response to the environmental and infectious selection pressures they continually face. Pigs are omnivores and their enteric system must logically be adapted to respond to the range of intestinal pathogens, and therefore defence mechanisms have developed to protect the host (pig) and maintain intestinal health. Nevertheless, and this will be discussed in more detail soon, the piglet is immunodeficient at birth and is highly dependent upon a supply of both specific and non-specific immune factors present in maternal colostrum and milk for immune protection, development and survival (Varley *et al.*, 1987). Therefore, development of immunocompetence is an absolute requirement for optimum growth and performance (Stokes *et al.*, 2004). Bailey *et al.* (2001) surmised that immunological development in the neonatal pig occurs as a balance between regulatory functions and effector functions, and that GIT integrity depends on the maintenance of this balance.

3. Neonatal immune function: general aspects

The immune system in the young pig comprises several organs (bone marrow, thymus, spleen, mesenteric lymph nodes) and several cell types (lymphocytes – specific immune recognition of foreign antigen; phagocytes – production of innate immunity) that recognise foreign antigens. The immune defence system has two 'arms' – the *innate* and the *acquired* (or *adaptive*). These will be discussed in more detail below, but basically, the innate immune system is thought to have evolved before the adaptive immune system, and hence has evolved also as the first line of defence against a pathogenic/antigenic challenge. Moreover, it is important to recognise that exposure to bacterial antigen is important in priming the immune system in the correct way and throughout life, to maintain a functional immune system (Kelly and Coutts, 2000; Kelly and King, 2001). The manipulation and (or) disruption of the microbiota and the immune system, such as during lactation and (or) at weaning, may have long-lasting effects on mucosal function (Pluske *et al.*, 2005). Bailey *et al.* (2001) suggested that the development of excessive regulatory or effector functions as a result of insults at weaning leaves the pig with a long-term inability to mount appropriate responses to mucosal antigens. Of equal importance is the type of bacteria that the intestine is exposed to, as different species and strains can exert very diverse effects on the gut, that range from beneficial to harmful (Umesaki *et al.*, 1999). Again, some of these aspects can be found in the paper by Gaskins (2008) in these proceedings.

4. Adaptive immune function

In neonates, the effector 'arm' of the adaptive immune system is functionally immature as developing lymphocytes undergo positive and negative selection in the thymus (Cahill *et al.*, 1999). Passive immunity via maternal nutrition, which provides constituents of both 'arms' of the immune system, makes available a number of defence factors such as immunoglobulins, lactoferrin, lysozyme and oligosaccharides, and may also influence the development of the systemic and mucosal adaptive immune system of neonates.

Adaptive immune responses are initiated following antigen uptake and presentation to T- and B-cells (Medzhitov and Janeway, 1997). Clonal expansion of T- and B-cell types requires specific signals from foreign or non-self antigens mostly from pathogens, which cause the production by lymphocytes of immunoglobulins. This 'arm' of the immune system is also influenced by the innate immune system, which in turn directs the adaptive responses to pathogens and other antigens (Kelly and King, 2001).

4.1. The gut-associated lymphoid system

The gut-associated lymphoid system (GALT) is intimate with the GIT epithelium and constitutes the largest mass of immune cells in the body (e.g. Rothkotter and Pabst, 1989). The GALT contains cells that function in antigen-specific immune responses, including the Peyer's patches (PP) of the small intestine that are discrete areas of organised lymphoid tissues in the lamina propria and submucosa with defined B and T lymphocyte areas characteristic of secondary lymphoid organs (Mowat and Viney, 1997). The ileal PP serves as a primary source of B cells in young pigs and consists of lymphoid follicles embedded in the lamina propria, so they cannot sample antigens directly from the gut lumen. In comparison, the jejunal PP follicles are found in a region of specialised dome epithelium, the follicle-associated epithelium (FAE). In addition to columnar epithelial cells, the FAE contains cuboidal epithelial cells referred to as microfold (M) cells, which lack a defined brush-border membrane, a thick glycocalyx, and an abundance of hydrolytic enzymes. The M cells are the only epithelial cells that endocytose and process luminal antigens for subsequent exposure to underlying B and T lymphocytes, and macrophages present in the M cell. The region underlying the PP dome harbours a variety of antigen-processing and antigen-presenting cells (APCs), and is a principal inductive site for immunity (Mowat and Viney, 1997). The uptake of antigens and other macromolecules involves the adherence of luminal material to the apical membrane of the M cell, and its subsequent capture and transcellular transport by endosomes (summarised by Dvorak *et al.*, 2006).

4.2. Acquisition of colostral antibodies

Low immunocompetency of the piglet at parturition coupled to insufficient intake of colostrum markedly increases the risk of piglet morbidity and mortality. Epitheliochorial placentation does not permit the transfer of maternal antibodies (predominately Immunoglobulin G) across the placenta to the foetus, meaning that the newborn piglet is essentially immunocompromised from the time it is born until it commences suckling and consumes colostral antibodies (Bourne, 1973). Very little antigen exposure occurs *in utero*, so at birth, the immune system of a healthy neonate, from an immunological standpoint, is naïve. During the birth process and early postnatal life, microbes from the mother and surrounding environment colonise the GIT of the infant. Exposure to this microbiota is a major predisposing factor in the anatomical and functional expansion of the intestinal immune system.

In the first weeks of life, as piglets expand the array of cell types needed to mount an adaptive immune response in reaction to environmental challenges, they receive protective immunoglobulins in the maternal colostrum and milk they consume at the udder. The level of protection given is limited by the quantity and quality of antibodies in colostrum and by the amount the neonate is able to consume and absorb (Jensen *et al.*, 2001; Le Dividich *et al.*, 2005). The predominant immunoglobulin isotype in colostrum is IgG and although maternal IgG is protective against many systemic pathogens, most pathogens encountered by the piglet are found at the mucosal surfaces where IgG antibodies are rare and largely ineffective (Gaskins, 1998). A second longer phase of passive protection, occurring as colostrum formation ends and lactation proceeds, results in IgG concentrations decreasing quickly as IgA becomes the major immunoglobulin in sow milk (e.g. Bourne, 1973; Klobasa *et al.*, 1986; Le Dividich *et al.*, 2005) (Figure 1). Maternal IgA provides short-term intestinal protection by inhibiting viral growth, inhibiting bacterial attachment, and by opsonising or lysing bacteria (Porter 1986; Gaskins 1998). Although suckling piglets receive partial protection against those antigens to which the sow has previously developed immunity, they have little or no protection against new infectious agents that may be introduced to rearing units (Kelly and King, 2001). This appears to especially be the case for piglets sucking from gilts or primiparous sows (Klobasa *et al.*, 1986).

The most abundantly produced immunoglobulin is IgA, which is synthesised by B2-type lymphocytes that are first exposed to antigens in intestinal PPs and then secreted mainly across mucous membranes (Kelly and King, 2001). Conventional immune responses leading to production of IgA involve two principal players, the T and B lymphocytes. Luminal antigens are transported through the specialised epithelial M cells overlying PPs, into an interfollicular area where they are presented by resident antigen presenting cells (macrophages and dendritic cells) to helper T (TH) lymphocytes. In turn, the TH cells secrete cytokines that stimulate B-lymphocytes that produce IgA. After leaving PPs and passing through the systemic circulation, IgA^+ lymphocytes migrate back

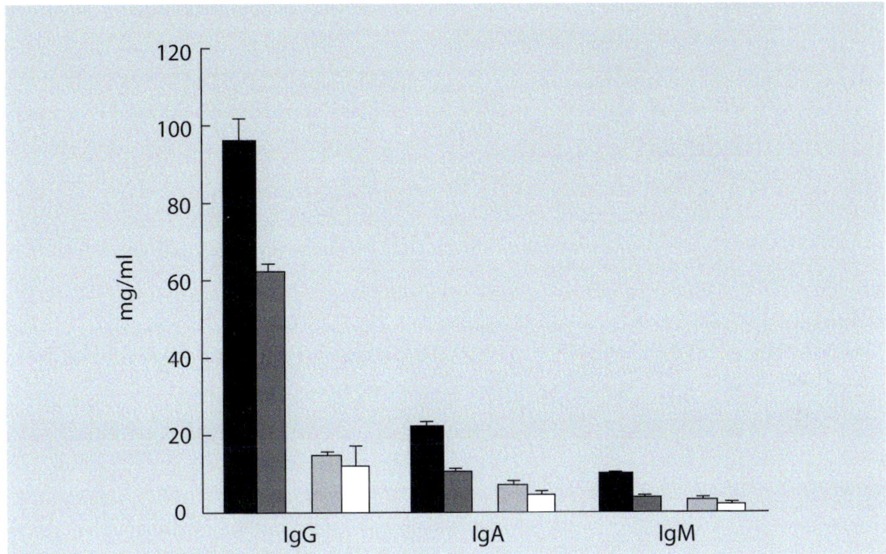

Figure 1. Concentrations of immunoglobulins in colostrum (before suckling) and milk (24 hours post-partum). Data (± SE) are adapted from Klobasa et al. *(1981; Colostrum [black], milk [dark grey]) and Curtis and Bourne (1971; colostrum [light grey], milk [white]).*

to the lamina propria where they differentiate into plasma cells capable of secreting large amounts of antibody (Kelly and King, 2001; Figure 2). Upon reintroduction of the antigen, plasma cells secrete antigen-specific IgA that is then transported back toward the intestinal lumen (see review by Gaskins, 1998).

Whilst newborn and suckling pigs possess some of the effector B-cell mechanisms to initiate immune responses, unfortunately they do not develop a fully functioning T-cell repertoire until the late sucking or early weaning periods (see Pabst and Rothkotter, 1989; Bianchi *et al.*, 1992; Zuckerman and Gaskins, 1996; Bailey *et al.*, 2001; Kelly and King, 2001; Thacker, 2003; Brown *et al.*, 2006). Numbers of both B and T lymphocytes present in the lamina propria virtually double during the first 4 weeks of life (summarised in Bailey *et al.*, 2001). Over the same period there occurs a marked change in the differentiation of the T-lymphocyte population as the piglet GIT develops (e.g. Rothkotter *et al.*, 1991, Gaskins 1998; Bailey *et al.*, 2001). Needless to say, the bacteria in the GIT play a most important role in the proliferation and development of these immune cell populations (Kelly and King, 2001).

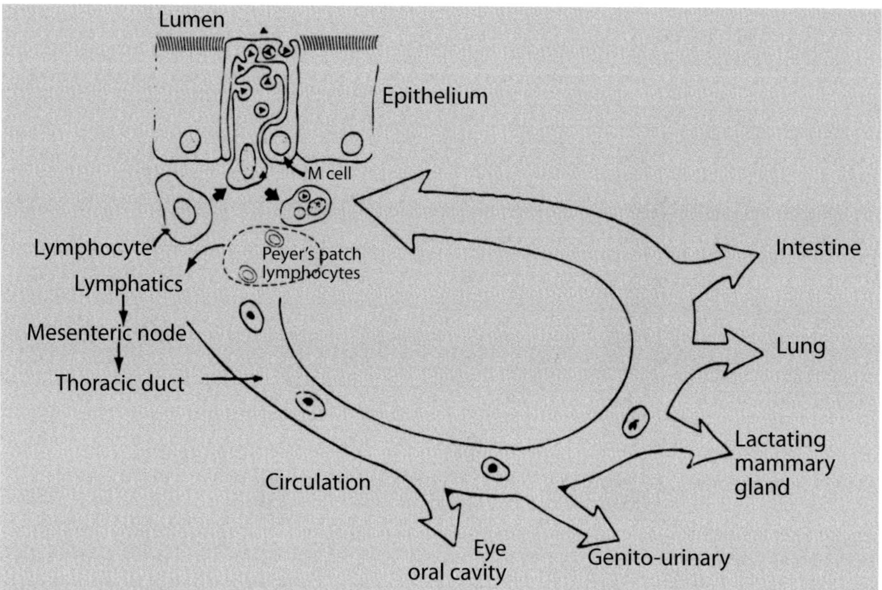

Figure 2. The intestinal contribution to the 'common mucosal immune system'. The secretory IgA system develops in Peyer's patches and IgA⁺ B lymphocytes then migrate back to all of the mucosal tissues (from Gaskins, 1998).

Unfortunately, current weaning ages occur at times when the young pig is still developing an immunological arsenal, and hence it is particularly vulnerable around this time.

4.3. Maternal nutrition and immune modulation

Kelly and Coutts (2000) overviewed the relationships between maternal nutrition and the 'education' of the immune system in the suckling piglet. It has long been established that differences exist in the growth, development and subsequent maturation between colostrum-fed and colostrum-deprived piglets, indicating the powerful effects the various components of colostrum, and to a lesser extent milk, from sows have on both the ecosystem and physical environment of the GIT. Kelly and Coutts (2000) described studies indicating that maternal milk can influence the maturation of the neonatal immune system, however they also indicated the contrary, whereby there are immunosuppressive effects of, for example, breast-feeding in humans, on development of active immune responses. The presence of large quantities of T lymphocytes and cytokines in mammalian milks will also have an effect on anti-microbial function and, in turn or independently of, immune system development. Furthermore, the apparent lack of inflammatory reactions in the gut against secretory IgA implicates the presence of anti-inflammatory compounds such as interleukin-10 (IL-10) and transforming growth factor-β (TGF-β) in milk (reviewed by Kelly and Coutts, 2000). Furthermore, Diaz *et al.* (2004) showed that the maternal adaptive immune system influences the pattern and abundance of bacteria in the GIT of their suckling young. Much of this work has obviously been conducted using mice and rats, and unfortunately only a small research effort has been directed towards the young pig. Nevertheless and in the context of pig production, these findings offer many exciting avenues for further research, and already some research supports this notion (e.g. Demecková *et al.*, 2002).

5. Innate immune function

The major function of the innate immune system is to act as first line of defence against infectious/pathogenic challenge to the animal. The major immune cells are macrophages, neutrophils and natural killer cells, and these recognise bacterial antigens via specific host recognition receptors (Kelly and King, 2001). The recognition of bacterial antigen causes an effector phase that activates the complement system, the production of chemokines, and the production of cytokines including IL-1, IL-6, interferon-gamma (IFN-γ), tumor necrosis factor-α (TNF-α), and reactive oxygen intermediates (Kelly and King, 2001).

Prominent host receptor systems are the toll-like receptors (TLRs). These trans-membrane receptors, which have a large extracellular leucine-rich repeat domain and a cytoplasmic domain, cause the activation of transcription factors, predominantly nuclear factor-kappa B (NF-κB) and AP-1 (see Kelly and King, 2001). The subsequent increase in expression and secretion of pro-inflammatory cytokines regulated by NF-κB, such as IL-1, IL-6 and IL-8, is important for the recruitment and activation of other cells of the mucosal immune system. Kelly and King (2001) and Stokes *et al.* (2004) describe the interaction between the TLRs and the luminal bacteria are described in more detail.

6. Weaning and the mucosal immune system

Weaning is characterised by significant nutritional, social and environmental changes that can impose a significant penalty on subsequent growth and production. A marked feature of weaning, irrespective of weaning age, is the transient decrease in macronutrient and micronutrient intake that occurs as pigs are switched abruptly from a mostly all-milk diet to a solid diet that differs in both the type of nutrients and the form of the nutrients (Pluske *et al.*, 1997). Despite the plethora of studies conducted in the past 40 years concerning nutrition and weaning of pigs under commercial farming conditions, there appears to have been very little research directed specifically towards the immune system, and particularly the mucosal immune system of the GIT. This would appear to be odd given that diet constituents become intimately associated with the mucosal epithelium in their passage through the GIT. However, and although not the subject of this paper, one of the most researched aberrant immune responses to antigens in the post-weaning diet is that caused specifically by feeding soy protein, and its purported effects on structure and function of the GIT and the immune system (e.g. Hampson, 1987; Bailey *et al.*, 1993; see review by Bailey *et al.*, 2001).

6.1. The post-weaned gastrointestinal tract: diet, inflammation and immunity

A heavily researched area in recent times deals with the effects of weaning, and the transient anorexia that occurs in conjunction with weaning, on GIT structure and function (summarised in Pluske *et al.*, 1997). In particular, emphasis on the roles of cytokines has received considerable attention. Cytokines are small peptide molecules that are important mediators in the regulation of the immune and inflammatory responses, and are believed to contribute to poor growth of immunologically challenged animals (Johnson, 1997). Although mostly derived from lymphocytes and macrophages, cytokines are also produced by epithelial cells, endothelial cells, and fibroblasts, which are effective sources and targets of cytokines (Pié *et al.*, 2004). Cytokines play a central role in immune cell response, but they also participate in the maintenance of tissue integrity. Changes in the cytokine network of the pig gut may be expected at weaning, because abrupt changes in dietary and environmental factors lead to important morphological and functional adaptations in the gut. Indeed, weaning-associated intestinal inflammation occurs in various animal species. For example, an increase of both $CD4^+$ (cluster of differentiation) and $CD8^+$-T lymphocyte subsets occurs as soon as 2 days after weaning in piglets (McCracken *et al.*, 1999).

Pié *et al.* (2004) demonstrated that weaning in piglets is associated with a transient inflammation of the GIT. Intestinal up-regulation of the pro-inflammatory cytokines IL-1ß, IL-6 and TNF-alpha mRNA occurred during the first 2 days after weaning but after this time, the mRNA level of most of these cytokines returned to pre-weaning levels. In a subsequent study, Pié *et al.*

(2007) examined whether feeding a diet containing fermentable carbohydrate sources (lactulose, inulin, sugar-beet pulp, and wheat starch) would influence proinflammatory cytokine expression in the GIT of newly-weaned piglets. These authors concluded that correlations between proinflammatory cytokines and the end-products of fermentation indicated that the regulation of cytokines may be linked with some of the fermentation end-products such as branched-chain fatty acids, which are in turn end-products of protein fermentation. Nevertheless, and as was reported earlier by McCracken *et al.* (1999), such changes were transient and the authors provided no evidence of any long-term negative effects of enhanced proinflammatory cytokine expression in the immediate post-weaning period.

7. Feed additives and GIT immunity

There are surprisingly few studies examining the roles *specifically* of feed additives/feed ingredients (aside from soy proteins, mentioned previously) on the immune system of the GIT in young pigs, although an increasing number of studies deriving predominately from Europe have occurred more recently in view of the ban on antibiotic feed additives in diets. The following sections discuss several feed additives/feed ingredients where these is some data on aspects of GIT immune function.

7.1. Yeast cell wall derivatives

Bio-Mos®, (Alltech Inc, USA), a mannan oligosaccharide derived from the cell wall of yeast (*Saccharomyces cerevisiae*) that consists of a mannan and a glucan component, has been shown to positively influence performance of weanling pigs (Miguel *et al.*, 2004). The positive actions of Bio-Mos® on performance are believed to occur through a combination of modification of the gut microbiota by blocking pathogen colonisation and inhibition of immune system activation (Davis *et al.*, 2004a,b). In young weaned pigs, Davis *et al.* (2004a) reported that Bio-Mos® altered the proliferation of lymphocytes isolated from peripheral blood. In a subsequent study, Davis *et al.* (2004b) reported that Bio-Mos®-supplemented pigs tended ($P<0.100$) to have a greater proportion of $CD14^+$ lamina propria leukocytes 19 days after weaning than pigs fed the diet lacking Bio-Mos®, indicating a greater proportion of macrophages present in the lamina propria of Bio-Mos®-fed pigs. Furthermore, Davis *et al.* (2004b) reported that pigs fed Bio-Mos® had a lower ($P<0.05$) ratio of $CD3^+CD4^+$: $CD3^+CD8^+$ T-lymphocytes on day 21 after weaning, indicating a greater proportion of $CD8^+$

T cells in the lamina propria. The lower $CD3^+CD4^+ : CD3^+CD8^+$ ratio found in Bio-Mos®-supplemented pigs concurs with changes seen after weaning in non-related, weaning-associated studies (McCracken *et al.*, 1999), and was surmised to represent the establishment of a more mature T-cell repertoire after weaning (Davis *et al.*, 2004b). However the precise aetiology of these changes could not be established. In addition, Davis *et al.* (2004b) found an increase in the percentage of lymphocytes and a decrease in the percentage of neutrophils in piglets fed Bio-Mos®, relative to pigs fed the basal diet. These authors postulated that the greater (P=0.140) lymphocyte:neutrophil ratio may be an indication that Bio-Mos® supplementation alleviates the alterations in immune function that cause an inflammatory reaction during the stress of weaning.

7.2. Spray-dried animal plasmas

Spray-dried animal plasma (protein) is used widely in the diets of weanling pigs to cause increases in food intake, growth rate and, potentially, food conversion efficiency. Dietary plasma protein stimulates growth rate largely by increasing food intake. This stimulation of food intake is a beneficial response because anorexia is an important factor limiting growth rate during the weaning transition (Jiang *et al.*, 2000). Spray-dried plasma protein is a complex mixture, containing fibrinogen immunoglobulin and albumin. The improvement in growth rate and food conversion seen in mice fed spray-dried plasma protein was reproduced by including only the immunoglobulin fraction of the product, and not the fibrinogen or albumin fractions (Godfredson-Kisic and Johnson, 1997). These data suggest that the immunoglobulin fraction of spray-dried plasma protein is responsible for the improved performance. Indeed, the growth response to spray-dried plasma protein is generally greater in pigs housed in a commercial nursery (and therefore presumably with greater pathogen exposure) than in pigs housed in a controlled experimental nursery environment (Coffey and Cromwell, 1995). Although it is unlikely that the immunoglobulins present in spray-dried plasma protein are absorbed across the intestinal wall in 3- to 4-wk old weaned pigs, they may affect the intestinal microflora and or the local intestinal immune responses associated with the weaning transition (Jiang *et al.*, 2000).

To investigate this further, Jiang *et al.* (2000) observed differences in total intestinal protein and DNA content in weaned piglets fed spray-dried plasma protein versus soy protein, and proposed this could reflect changes in cellularity of the lamina propria as well as the epithelial cell layer. These authors also observed a significant increase in total blood leukocyte numbers during the 16-day feeding period, suggestive of a systemic proinflammatory response, but found no differences among the dietary groups. In addition, Jiang *et al.* (2000) found that the intestinal intravillus lamina propria cell density, specifically lymphocytes, increased during the 16-day period, and this increase in cell density may have been a consequence of increased local intestinal inflammation. Lamina propria cell density was significantly lower in pigs fed plasma protein than in pigs fed soy protein, leading the authors to speculate that dietary plasma protein may suppress the local intestinal proinflammatory response associated with weaning and thereby reduce leukocytic infiltration into the mucosal lamina propria.

7.3. Plant extracts

A replacement touted for antibiotic feed additives for newly-weaned pigs is essential oils. A considerable body of information, much of it equivocal, has now been established investigating the efficacy of essential oils/plant extracts on production and GIT health in the young, newly-weaned pig. Plant extracts are the ingredients of many commercial preparations currently used in pig production and present an array of purported beneficial effects. Many studies have been conducted, however one study by Manzanilla *et al.* (2006) reported that a mixture of 5% (wt/wt) carvacrol (from *Origanun* spp.), 3% cinnamaldehyde (from *Cinnamonum* spp.) and 2% capsicum oleoresin (from *Capsicum annum*) fed to weaner pigs (0.03% of the diet) decreased the number of intraepithelial lymphocytes in the jejunum and ileum and increased lymphocytes in the colon. The true significance of such results from a production perspective was difficult to ascertain, particularly in light of the lack of treatment differences in production against the control diet. Nevertheless, a companion paper by Castillo *et al.* (2006) reported changes in the ecological structure and metabolic activity of the microbial ecosystem of the GIT in response to the plant extract combination that, in turn, could have influenced immune cell populations.

7.4. Probiotics

As discussed previously, bacterial colonisation of the GIT influences the function of immune cells belonging to the GALT and can affect the systemic immune system, and a number of studies have reported immune-stimulating effects of different bacterial species. It has also been shown that bacterial colonisation contributes to the induction and maintenance of immunological tolerance against nutritional antigens (Kelly and King, 2001). The beneficial effects of bacteria on the immune system have been proposed as one basis supporting the use of probiotic bacteria as an alternative to antibiotics in improving animal health and protection against infectious agents (e.g. Schiffrin and Blum, 2002). For example, lactic acid bacteria have been found to increase the total amount of intestinal IgA (Vitini *et al.*, 2000).

A growing number of studies have been conducted now in pigs, and to review all of these is outside the scope of this paper. However, in one study in sows and piglets that I wish to allude to, Scharek *et al.* (2005) examined the effects of the probiotic bacterium *Enterococcus faecium* SF68 on the immune system and the intestinal colonisation of pigs. Mucosal immunity of the developing piglets was monitored by isolation and detection of intestinal lymphocyte cell populations from the proximal jejunal epithelium and the continuous PP by the use of flow cytometry. Levels of intestinal IgA in both groups of piglets were compared, as well as total IgG in the serum of sows and piglets. Faeces of the sows and intestinal contents of the piglets were taken for determination of total anaerobe and coliform bacterial counts in both probiotic and control groups. Villus length and depth of the crypts were measured in the jejunum of sacrificed piglets.

Scharek *et al.* (2005) reported that total serum IgG of the sows was unaffected. Piglets of both groups showed similar IgG levels up to 5 weeks after birth with a slight tendency toward lower values in the probiotic group. At an age of 8 weeks the total IgG levels of the probiotic animals were significantly lower ($P<0.01$). No differences were observed in the populations of $CD4^+$ and $CD8^+$ T cells in the PP, however levels of cytotoxic T cells ($CD8^+$) in the jejunal epithelium of piglets of the probiotic group were reduced. Jejunal crypt depth and villous height were similar in both groups, suggesting the relative T-cell population differences were not due to alterations in the epithelial cell numbers. The total anaerobe and coliform bacterial populations were not affected by the probiotic treatment, either in sows or in the piglets, although the authors found a decrease in the frequency of β-haemolytic and O141 serovars of *Escherichia coli* in the intestinal contents of probiotic piglets, suggesting an explanation for the reduction in cytotoxic T-cell populations.

8. Conclusions

The interactions between commensal and pathogenic bacteria, the host and nutrition GIT are crucial for the development and expansion of the immune system of the GIT. Changes in diet, including the loss of protective immunity contained in sows' milk, associated with weaning causes disturbances in the GIT that alter how the immune system subsequently processes bacterial and dietary antigens (Kelly and King, 2001). Dietary manipulation is seen as a means of possible manipulation to induce a more 'favourable' education of the immune response, however the vast number of interactions that occur in the GIT between nutrition, the host and the commensal and pathogenic biota make this an interesting challenge.

References

Bailey, M., Miller, B.G., Telemo, E., Stokes, C.R. and Bourne, F.J. (1993). Specific immunological unresponsiveness following active primary responses to proteins in the weaning diet of piglets. *International Archives in Allergy and Immunology* **101:** 266-271.

Bailey, M., Plunkett, F.J., Rothkotter, H-J, Vega-Lopez, M.A., Haverson, K. and Stokes, C.R. (2001). Regulation of mucosal immune responses in effector sites. *Proceedings of the Nutrition Society* **60:** 427-435.

Bianchi, A.T.J., Zwart, R.J., Jeurissen, S.H.M. and Moonenleusen, H.W.M. (1992). Development of the B-cell and T-cell compartments in porcine lymphoid organs from birth to adult life – an immunohistological approach. *Veterinary Immunology and Immunopathology* **33**: 201-221.

Brown, D.C., Maxwell, C.V., Erf, G.F., Davis, M.E., Singh, S. and Johnson, Z.B. (2006). Ontogeny of T lymphocytes and intestinal morphological characteristics in neonatal pigs at different ages in the postnatal period. *Journal of Animal Science* **84:** 567-578.

Bourne, F.J. (1973). The immunoglobulin system of the young pig. *Proceedings of the Nutrition Society* **32:** 205-215.

Cahill, R.N.P., Kimpton, W.G., Washington, E.A., Holder, J.E. and Cunningham, C.P. (1999). The ontogeny of T cell recirculation during fetal life. *Seminars in Immunology* **11:** 105-114.

Castillo, M., Martín-Orúe, S.M., Roca, M., Manzanilla, E.G., Badiola, I., Perez, J.F. and Gasa, J. (2006). The response of gastrointestinal microbiota to avilamycin, butyrate, and plant extracts in early-weaned pigs. *Journal of Animal Science* **84:** 2725-2734.

Coffey R.D. and Cromwell G.L. (1995). The impact of environment and antimicrobial agents on the growth response of early-weaned pigs to spray-dried porcine plasma. *Journal of Animal Science* **73:** 2532-2539.

Curtis, J. and Bourne, F.J. (1971). Immunoglobulin quantitation in sow serum, colostrum and milk and the serum of young pigs. *Biochimica Biophysica Acta* **236:** 319-322.

Demecková, V., Kelly, D., Coutts, A.G.P., Brooks, P.H. and Campbell, A. (2002). The effect of fermented liquid feeding on the faecal microbiology and colostrum quality of farrowing sows. *International Journal of Food Microbiology* **79:** 85-97.

Davis, M.E., Brown, D.C., Maxwell, C.V., Johnson, Z.B., Kegley, E.B. and. Dvorak, R.A. (2004a). Effect of phosphorylated mannans and pharmacological additions of zinc oxide on growth and immunocompetence of weanling pigs. *Journal of Animal Science* **82:** 581-587.

Davis, M.E., Maxwell, C.V., Erf, G.F., Brown and Wistuba, T.J. (2004b). Dietary supplementation with phosphorylated mannans improves growth response and modulates immune function of weanling pigs. *Journal of Animal Science* **82:** 1882-1891.

Diaz, R.L., Hoang, L., Wang, J., Vela, J.L., Jenkins, S., Aranda, R. and Martin, M.G. (2004). Maternal adaptive immunity influences the intestinal microflora of suckling mice. *Journal of Nutrition* **134:** 2359-2364.

Dvorak, C.M.T., Hirsch, G.N., Hyland, K.A., Hendrickson, J.A., Thompson, B.S., Rutherford, M.S. and Murtaugh, M.P. (2006). Genomic dissection of mucosal immunobiology in the porcine small intestine. *Physiological Genomics* **28:** 5-14.

Gaskins, H.R. (1998). Immunological development and mucosal defence in the pig intestine. In: *Progress in Pig Science* (Eds. J. Wiseman, M.A. Varley and J.P. Chadwick). Nottingham University Press, Nottingham, UK. pp. 81-101.

Gaskins, H.R. (2008). Host and intestinal microbiota negotiations in the context of animal growth efficiency. In: *Gut efficiency; the key ingredient in pig and poultry production* (Eds. J.A. Taylor-Pickard and P. Spring). Wageningen Academic Publishers, Wageningen, The Netherlands. pp. 29-37.

Godfredson-Kisic J.A. and Johnson D.E. (1997). A bioassay used to identify the active fraction of spray-dried porcine plasma. *Journal of Animal Science* **75:** 195(Abs.)

Hampson, D.J. (1987). Dietary influences on porcine postweaning diarrhoea. In: *Manipulating Pig Production* (Eds. J.L. Barnett, E.S. Batterham, G.M. Cronin, C. Hansen, P.H. Hemsworth, P.E. Hughes, N.E. Johnston and R.H. King). Australasian Pig Science Association, Werribee, Victoria, Australia. pp. 202-214.

Jensen, A.R., Elnif, J., Burrin, D.G. and Sangild, P.T. (2001). Development of intestinal immunoglobulin absorption and enzyme activities in neonatal pigs is diet dependent. *Journal of Nutrition* **131:** 3259-3265.

Jiang, R., Chang, X., Stoll, B., Ellis, K.J., Shypailo, R.J., Weaver, E., Campbell, J. and Burrin, D.G. (2000). Dietary plasma protein is used more efficiently than extruded soy protein for lean tissue growth in early-weaned pigs. *Journal of Nutrition* **130:** 2016-2019.

Johnson, R.W. (1997). Inhibition of growth by pro-inflammatory cytokines: An integrated view. *Journal of Animal Science* **75:** 1244-1255.

Kelly, D. and Conway, S. (2005). Bacterial modulation of mucosal innate immunity. *Molecular Immunology* **42:** 895-901.

Kelly, D., and Coutts, A.G.P. (2000). Early nutrition and the development of immune function in the neonate. *Proceedings of the Nutrition Society* **59:** 177-185.

Kelly, D. and King, T.P. (2001). A review – Luminal bacteria and regulation of gut function and immunity. In: *Manipulating Pig Production VIII* (Ed. P.D. Cranwell). Australasian Pig Science Association, Werribee, Victoria, Australia. pp. 263-276.

Klobasa, F., Butler, J.E., Werhahn, E. and Habe, F. (1986). Maternal-neonatal immunoregulation in swine. II. Influence of multiparity on *de novo* immunoglobulin synthesis by piglets. *Veterinary Immunology and Immunopathology* **11:** 149-159.

Le Dividich, J., Rooke, J.A. and Herpin, P. (2005). Nutritional and immunological importance of colostrum for the new-born pig. *Journal of Agricultural Science* **143:** 469-485.

Manzanilla, E.G., Nofrarias, M., Anguita, M., Castillo, M., Perez, J.F., Martin-Orue, S.M., Kamel, C. and Gasa, J. (2006). Effects of butyrate, avilamycin, and a plant extract combination on the intestinal equilibrium of early-weaned pigs. *Journal of Animal Science* **84:** 2743-2751.

McCracken, B.A., Spurlock, M.E., Roos, M.A., Zuckermann, F.A. and Gaskins, H.R. (1999). Weaning anorexia may contribute to local inflammation in the piglet small intestine. *Journal of Nutrition* **129:** 613-619.

Medzhitov, R. and Janeway, C.A. (1997). Innate immunity: the virtues of a nonclonal system of recognition. *Cell* **91**: 295-298.

Miguel, J.C., Rodriguez-Zas, S.L. and Pettigrew, J.E. (2004). Efficacy of a mannan oligosaccharide (Bio-Mos®) for improving nursery pig performance. *Journal of Swine Health and Production* **12**: 296-307.

Mowat, A.M. and Viney, J.L. (1997). The anatomical basis of intestinal immunity. *Immunological Reviews* **156:** 145-166.

Pabst, R. and Rothkotter, H.J. (1989). Postnatal development of lymphocyte subsets in different compartments of the small intestine of piglets. *Veterinary Immunology and Immunopathology* **72:** 167-173.

Pié, S., Awati, A., Vida, S., Falluel, I., Williams, B.A. and Oswald, I.P. (2007). Effects of added fermentable carbohydrates in the diet on intestinal proinflammatory cytokine-specific mRNA content in weaning piglets. *Journal of Animal Science* **85:** 673-683.

Pié, S., Lalles, J.P., Blazy, F., Laffitte, J., Seve, B. and Oswald, I.P. (2004). Weaning is associated with an upregulation of expression of inflammatory cytokines in the intestine of piglets. *Journal of Nutrition* **134:** 641-647.

Pluske, J.R., Williams, I.H. and Hampson, D.J. (1997). Factors influencing the structure and function of the small intestine in the weaned pig: a review. *Livestock Production Science* **51:** 215-236.

Pluske, J.R., Payne, H.G., Williams, I.H. and Mullan, B.P. (2005). Early feeding for lifetime performance of pigs. In: *Recent Advances in Animal Nutrition in Australia Volume 15* (Eds. P.B. Cronje and N. Richards, eds.). Animal Science, University of New England, Armidale, NSW. pp. 171-181.

Porter, P. (1986). Immune System. In: *Diseases of Swine* (Ed. A.D. Leman). Iowa University Press. Iowa State, Ames, USA. pp. 44-57.

Rothkotter, H.J. and Pabst, R. (1989). Lymphocyte subsets in jejunal and ileal Peyer's patches of normal and gnotobiotic minipigs. *Immunology* **67:** 103-108.

Rothkotter, H.J., Ulbrich, H. and Pabst, R. (1991). The postnatal development of gut lamina propria lymphocytes: Number proliferator and T and B cell subsets in conventional and germ-free pigs. *Pediatric Research* **29:** 237-242.

Rowlands, B.J. and Gardiner, K.R. (1998). Nutritional modulation of gut inflammation. *Proceedings of the Nutrition Society* **57:** 395-401.

Scharek, L., Guth, J., Reiter, K., Weyrauch, K.D., Taras, D., Schwerk, P., Schierack, P., Schmidt, M.F.G., Wieler, L.H. and Tedin. K. (2005). Influence of a probiotic *Enterococcus faecium* strain on development of the immune system of sows and piglets. *Veterinary Immunology and Immunopathology* **105:** 151-161.

Schiffrin, L. and Blum, S. (2002). Interactions between the microbiota and the intestinal mucosa. *European Journal of Clinical Nutrition* **56 (Suppl. 3):** S60-S64.

Stokes, C.R., Bailey, M., Haverson, K., Harris, C., Jones, P., Inman, C., Pie, S., Oswald, I.P., Williams, B.A., Akkermans, A.D.L., Sowa, E., Rothkotter, H.-J. and Miller, B.G. (2004). Postnatal development of intestinal immune system in piglets: implication for the process of weaning. *Animal Research* **53:** 325-334

Thacker, E.L. (2003). Immunology – the innate immune system. *The Pig Journal* **52:** 111-123.

Umesaki, Y., Setoyama, H., Matsumoto, S., Imaoka, A., and Itoh, K. (1999). Differential roles of segmented filamentous bacteria and clostridia in development of the intestinal immune system. *Infection and Immunity* **67**: 3504-3511.

Van Leeuwen, P.A.M., Boermeester, M.A., Houdijk, A.P.J., Ferwarda. C.C., Cuesta, M.A., Meyer, S., and Wesdorp, R.I.C. (1994). Clinical significance of transloaction. *Gut* **35 (Suppl. 1):** S28-S34.

Varley, M.A., Wilkinson, R.G. and Maitland, A. (1987). Artificial rearing of piglets: The effects of colostrum on survival and plasma concentrations of IgG. *British Veterinary Journal* **143:** 369-378.

Vitini, E., Alvarez, S., Medina, M., Medici, M., De Budeguer, M.V. and Perdign, G. (2000). Gut mucosal immunostimulation by lactic acid bacteria. *Biocell* **24:** 223-232.

Zuckerman, F.A. and Gaskins, H.R. (1996). Distribution of porcine CD4/CD8 double-positive lymphocytes in mucosa-associated lymphoid tissues. *Immunology* **87:** 493-499.

Pig health and the modern genotype: implications for performance and profitability

Steven McOrist
University of Nottingham, School of Veterinary Medicine and Science, Sutton Bonington, LE12 5RD, United Kingdom

1. Introduction

The raising of pigs in close association with their human owners was the norm until processes of intensification were developed in the 1960's in Europe and the Americas; but these farms still predominate in much of Asia. Development of extensive, 'organic' farming for niche markets in the west is, in many ways, a throw-back to the pre-intensive era. In these farms, numerous major endemic diseases thrive, such as the respiratory complexes, swine dysentery, salmonellosis and intestinal parasitism. Intensification processes include housing of specific age groups into separate larger units composed of breeding, nursery or fattening pigs, and use of formulated feeds, vaccines and medications. While the broader benefits of intensification include reductions in the major endemic diseases and smaller land usage for food production, complex alterations in disease patterns are usually noted, with apparent susceptibility to 'new' agents, such as *Haemophilus parasuis*, *Mycoplasma hyopneumoniae* and *Lawsonia intracellularis*. Modern western genotypes show high levels of susceptibility to a range of both the older and newer endemic diseases. The poor 'survivability' of modern synthetic lines has been identified following a long period of selection for production traits such as feed conversion and carcass quality. This link between genotype and health is being addressed in many recent commercial breeding programs.

Most pigs in the world are raised in farms in China and south-east Asia and many improved farms in that region boast imported western genotypes. Their swine production continues to move ahead in terms of consolidation, expertise and production levels. China currently has 1.3 billion consumers for 620 million slaughter pigs, produced from 50 million sows. Pig raising in Asia is usually split into 3 distinct segments: Traditional back-yard producers operating with 1 to 10 sows, small family producers with an average herd size of 40 sows and developing integrators with commercial or intensive farms (defined as more than 50 sows per farm), which are basically the western pig farming model. The latter are quickly increasing in number and overall integration throughout the region, particularly around major expanding cities such as Beijing (population 14m), Shanghai (population 17m) and Guangzhou (population 12m), where urbanisation (the marked shift in population from rural areas to the cities) is most active. In some of these peri-urban areas, the commercial farm segment is considered 60 to 80% of pig populations.

These intensification processes towards the western model include housing of specific age groups into separate larger units composed of breeding, nursery or fattening pigs. These farms may also have dedicated breeder pig suppliers, either western or local genotypes; complex commercial feed suppliers and may use off-site, contractor finisher farms. Pig housing, vaccinations, antibiotic usage, all-in, all-out and disinfection procedures are often improved. The Wens Animal Husbandry Co., based in Guangdong is regarded as China's largest integrated pig company, with 110,000 sows. The Charoen Pokphand group operates throughout South-East Asia, based in Bangkok, and has 100,000 sows, and many other major operations are developing.

The key broader benefits of swine farm intensification include more effective land usage for food production – China has only 7% of the world's cultivable land, but has 22% of the world's population. Development of an efficient farm sector also addresses two other main community policies – food security for the entire population and increasing incomes in rural areas to attempt to offset or arrest urbanisation. Agriculture remains an important part of Asian economies; producing 15% of GDP and accounting for 40% of employment in China. There is therefore still considerable support for backyard farms, where small numbers of pigs are fed crop residues, table scraps and forage in simple housing. This type of farm probably still represents 70 to 80% of the total number of pigs raised in China and several other south-east Asian countries. These pigs add value to subsistence farming, as over 80% of these household farms have less than 0.6 hectare – not enough to support a family by crop production alone. In this system, crop production and animal raising are complementary and the low-cost pigs are viewed as a 'savings bank'.

Despite this, urbanisation continues at a rapid pace in China and throughout Asia. On average, families that move to the city will show a considerable rise in income, perhaps joining the manufacturing workforce. Given the scale of the population in China, this translates to a considerable growth in urban, middle class families in places like Shanghai or Beijing. Figure 1 illustrates the creation of an extra 40 million middle class Chinese households in the past

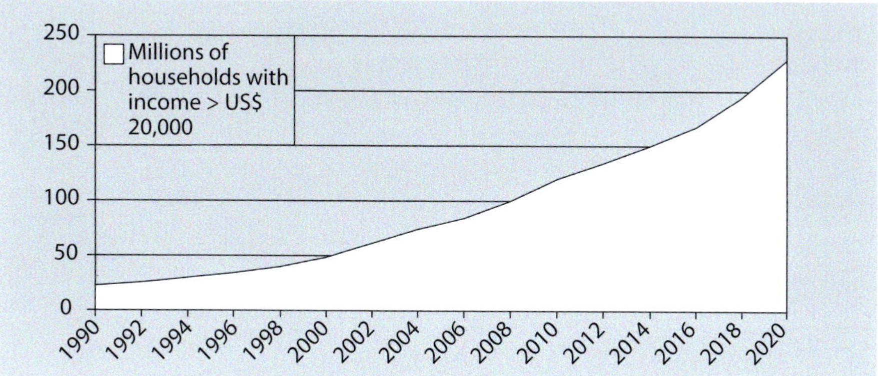

Figure 1. The rapid and projected rise over time of the Chinese middle classes is illustrated by an estimation of the total number of households with 'western' levels of income, defined as at least US$ 20,000 per year. It is expected that as the numbers of these consumers with extra disposable income increases, that consumption of dietary protein will also increase.

decade, a trend which is predicted to continue. These newly-enriched neo-urban families will typically purchase more meat protein. An average Chinese city population growth of 4% per year will directly lead to a similar increase in pork sales. The Chinese cultural preference for pork over other forms of meat has further translated this into an increased proportion of pork purchased as a percentage of the increased overall meat purchased, see Figure 2. Based on income growth alone, pork consumption will grow by a further 3% per year in urban areas (total 7%) and 1.5 to 2% in rural areas in China. Provinces of China such as Hong Kong SAR that already have western levels of wealth show pork consumption levels of nearly 60 kg per person per year, indicating that even more growth may occur.

The continued expansion of the industry (Figure 3) and the inherent supply-demand risks in the pig industry has led to further state interventions being considered and even encouraged by some policy groups. Data on the pig industry outputs/prices, etc. is limited in China, making risk assessment and price control difficult, even with an interventionist policy. Farmer organisations are poorly formed, with no equivalent of the NPPC or similar bodies. Related policy ideas have included imposition of quotas on the numbers of sows each farm is allowed; collection of restaurant waste or other industrial by-products from cities for feeding to pig farms. One area that remains greatly under-explored in the expansion of the industry in China is swine breeding – regional

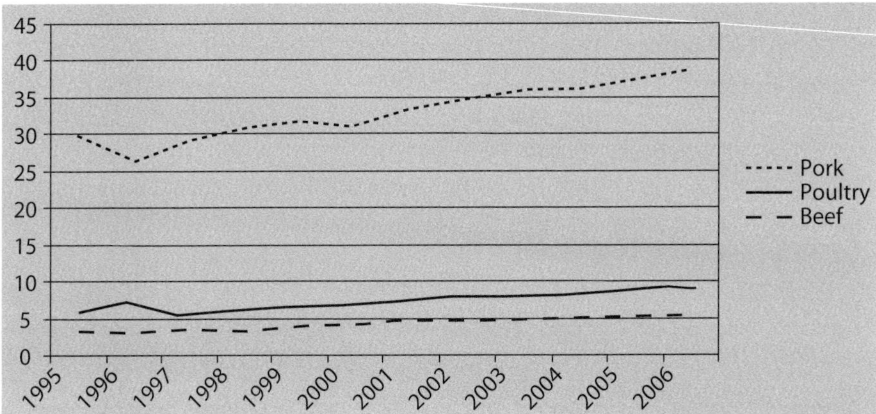

Figure 2. The levels of meat consumption in China are illustrated in numbers of kg consumed per person per year. Two factors are evident – as the levels of income have risen, the amount of protein meat consumed also rises. This rise in per capita meat consumption is separate and incremental to the rise in total meat consumed in China that would be predicted from increased population alone. Secondly, the rise in consumption of pork is greater than that for other meats indicating a clear preference for fresh pork products among Asian consumers. This has clear implications for pork production in China, especially as China restricts imports of pork.

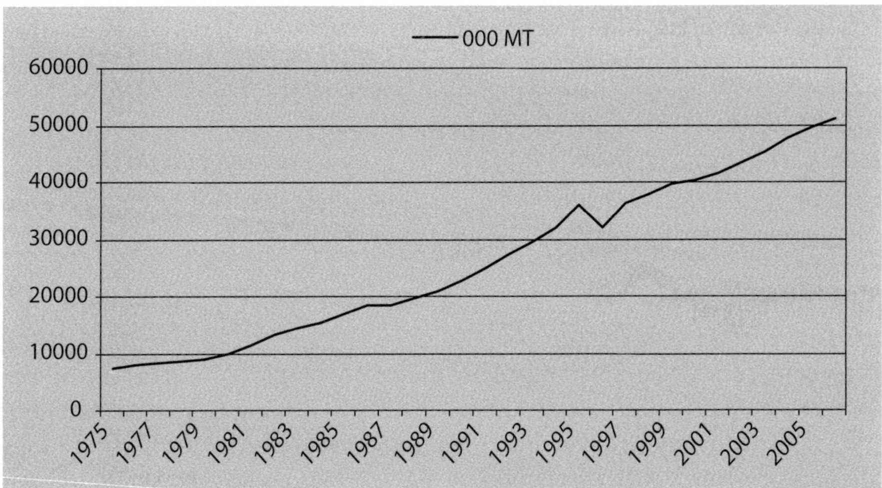

Figure 3. The levels of pig production in China are illustrated by the rise in the number of metric tonnes produced in China over time. Chinese pork production is growing steadily, with occasional supply-demand issues, exacerbated by the large number of small farms and lack of imports.

breeding centres have limited European or local X European stock. There are therefore few farm pigs with the improved feed conversion characters, typical of western pig breeding advances in the past decade. Artificial insemination from off-site, dedicated boar studs is largely unavailable.

While pig farms are being developed all over China, there were some extra increases in the Northern provinces, due to enhanced proximity to local Chinese corn supplies. However these Northern provinces (Jilin, Shandong etc) suffer from lack of technical expertise and lack of easy access for their pork products to the major markets, such as Beijing, Shanghai and Guangzhou. There is also currently a rapid rise in corn usage for biofuel production in Northern China, diverting animal feed into ethanol production, with consequent availability and price issues, identical to those occurring in North America. This suggested 'northern shift' has therefore stalled and most recent pig farm consolidation continues to occur in the southern and eastern coastal belt.

Manufactured commercial feeds are now widely used and the actual diet content is usually a standard corn-soy base diet. Feed normally arrives on farm in bags, which allows accurate data on feed consumption and costs. Even backyard farms typically use some manufactured feed as supplement. Most commercial pigs are fed and managed under normal western-style finisher pig conditions, except that they may be limit-fed. This limit feeding of pigs is commonly used to allow farmers to keep feed costs lower, improve leanness and to juggle pig outputs to perhaps wait for better prices. On some farms, high feed prices and market conditions meant that pigs targeted for only a 100 kg liveweight may not reach it until 24 or more weeks-old, even with western origin 'pink' pigs. The use of western genotypes that have been carefully bred for maximum daily gain and feed conversion has yet to find full acceptance in Asia, partly because limit-feeding reduces the impact of the genotype.

2. Sources of pig genotypes in Asia

Most commercial farms with western pigs derive their key breeding stock from provincial swine breeding centres, either Government or privately run. These centres have usually had on-going imports of western breeding stock in air-freighted batches of 40 to 100 sows. The largest one is the state-backed China National Animal Breeding Stock Corporation based in Beijing. But all provinces have their own swine breeding centre: typical examples include the Yisheng centre with 3,000 sows located in Yentai, Shandong, which imported

Pietrain and Large Whites from North America and the Guoshou development Co. with 2,000 sows in Xiamen, Fujian province, which imported pigs from nearby Taiwan. Overseas breeding companies have a small presence in China; PIC has made considerable efforts to set up 2 separate nucleus herds, and a new multiplier herd in Hubei, with well-run facilities and a range of PIC line pigs. Topigs and Hypor also have nucleus herd operations in China. The Thai Charoen Pokphand swine farming group has set up a large number of breeder herd start-up operations in China and Vietnam over the past 20 years, typically as joint ventures with local groups. Pigs for these farms have usually originated from the Thai-based grandparent CP line 40 or 51, which are based on Large White/Landrace crosses.

Again, the size of the local fatty breed market should not be underestimated. Some larger breeder operations exist, which carry the most popular breeds. For example, the Zhejiang centre has 400 Jinhua sows; the Suzhou City centre offers both meat breed sows, such as SuTai and mothering sow breeds such as the Meischan and Fengjing. In these and many more centres, local breed sows are cross-bred to form new lines such as a Tai Hu/Duroc cross production pig line.

Live on-farm boars remain popular due to the difficulties with establishing a boar stud program with a proper distribution network of semen supplies. Unlike Thailand, semen imports are rare in China. Most commercial farms make a considerable effort to purchase quality boars from the provincial breeding centres, with occasional live boar auctions occurring, for example at the Guangzhou swine breeding centre.

3. Disease patterns

Alterations in disease patterns due to intensification in Asia have been reviewed elsewhere by Ranald Cameron (2000). Among the many complex changes in disease transmission with increasing intensification, the more limited contact between sows and their children may lead to reduced early transmission of some agents, with consequent susceptibility to these agents if introduced to them at a later age. For some well-adapted porcine agents, such as *Haemophilus parasuis*, *Mycoplasma hyopneumoniae* and *Lawsonia intracellularis*, this later contact can lead to enhanced clinical signs.

On backyard farms in South-East Asia, old favourites such as foot and mouth disease (FMD) and classical swine fever (CSF) remain very common, with little biosecurity and few vaccinations occurring, due to the low-cost business model. These pigs and other infected livestock (such as feral goats) represent a clear danger for clean commercial and breeder herds. The Government-controlled CAHIC vaccine group has a range of modern factories around China. These can supply a range of vaccines including FMD and CSF. There are also several smaller local vaccine companies in China producing PRRS and other vaccines. Supply, potency, handling and storage of locally produced vaccines all remain important issues. The government has made considerable strides to improve registration procedures for western origin vaccines. Many western-origin swine vaccines from Merial or Boehringer are now centrally registered and freely available for use. PRRS vaccines have proved especially popular. However, the price of vaccines (both imported and local) means that they often remain limited in use to more progressive farms for swine farm improvements. Registration of foreign-origin FMD vaccines remains blocked in China. In other countries, such as Thailand, imported vaccines are widely available.

3. Conclusions

Intensification processes include housing of specific age groups into separate larger units composed of breeding, nursery or fattening pigs, and use of formulated feeds, vaccines and medications. Modern western genotypes show high levels of susceptibility to a range of both the older and newer endemic diseases. Most pigs in the world are raised in farms in China and south-east Asia and many improved farms in that region boast imported western genotypes. China currently has 1.3 billion consumers for 620 million slaughter pigs, produced from 50 million sows. Pig raising in Asia is usually split into 3 distinct segments: Traditional back-yard producers operating with 1 to 10 sows, small family producers with an average herd size of 40 sows and developing integrators with commercial or intensive farms (defined as more than 50 sows per farm), which are basically the western pig farming model. In some of these peri-urban areas, the commercial farm segment is considered 60 to 80% of pig populations.

These intensification processes towards the western model include housing of specific age groups into separate larger units composed of breeding, nursery or fattening pigs. These farms may also have dedicated breeder pig suppliers, either western or local genotypes; complex commercial feed suppliers and may use off-site, contractor finisher farms. The Wens Animal Husbandry Co., based in Guangdong is regarded as China's largest integrated pig company, with 110,000 sows. The key broader benefits of swine farm intensification include more effective land usage for food production – China has only 7% of the world's cultivable land, but has 22% of the world's population. This type of farm probably still represents 70 to 80% of the total number of pigs raised in China and several other south-east Asian countries. There are therefore few farm pigs with the improved feed conversion characters, typical of western pig breeding advances in the past decade. Most commercial farms with western pigs derive their key breeding stock from provincial swine breeding centres, either Government or privately run. Unlike Thailand, semen imports are rare in China. Most commercial farms make a considerable effort to purchase quality boars from the provincial breeding centres, with occasional live boar auctions occurring, for example at the Guangzhou swine breeding centre. There are also several smaller local vaccine companies in China producing PRRS and other vaccines. Many small and large farms retain fatty breed pigs for local and wider markets of fresh pork and specialised products such as Jinhua hams and Xiang pigs. Poor performance due to major disease outbreaks remains an important issue throughout the Asian pig farming industry.

References

Cameron, R.D.A. (2000). A review of the industrialisation of pig production worldwide with particular reference to the Asian region. Focus is on clarifying the animal and human health risks and reviewing the Area Wide Integration concept of specialised crop and livestock activities. FAO: http://www.fao.org/ag/againfo/resources/en/publications/agapubs/awi_concept_pig_product.pdf

The role of fibre in piglet gut health

Knud Erik Bach Knudsen, Helle Nygaard Lærke and Mette Skou Hedemann
University of Aarhus, Faculty of Agricultural Sciences, Department of Animal Health, Welfare and Nutrition, Blichers Allé 20, DK-8830 Tjele, Denmark

1. Introduction

Although the pig industry is among the most technologically advanced of all the animal industries the mortality of newborn piglets is still quite high with 15-20% of all pigs born alive being lost before delivered for slaughter. The critical periods are the neonatal phase (the first days after birth), the weaning period (when weaning at 4 weeks of age the first two weeks) and the first weeks after the pigs are being transferred to the feeding house. The overall mortality rate in the pig industry has not changed substantially in recent years, and is considerably higher than for other farm animals.

The problems that confront the piglets at weaning are unique and not experienced in other phases of the pigs growth: (1) the diet changes from liquid sow's milk to solid feed with a more complex structure, (2) the piglets are mixed and moved and there are changes in the environmental temperature, (3) there are marked changes in the structure and function of the small intestine that happens within 24 h of weaning, and (4) there are frequently outbreaks of diarrhoea due to proliferation of enterotoxigenic bacteria (mainly *Escherichia coli*) in the small intestine and/or fermentation of less digestible nutrients in the large intestine (Pluske *et al.*, 1995, 1997; Hampson *et al.*, 1999). The combined effect of these changes at weaning is that piglets generally display weight loss or poor growth, low levels of voluntary feed intake (VFI) and, in some instances, diarrhoea, morbidity and death (Hampson and Kidder, 1986). Antibiotics are the main tool to prevent or to treat such illness, but in-feed antibiotics also accelerate the growth of otherwise healthy animals (Armstrong, 1986). Unfortunately, the risk associated with long term used of excessive antibiotics for veterinary purposes may eventually result in a selection for the survival of resistant bacterial species or strains. Genes encoding for this resistance can be transferred to other formerly susceptible bacteria, thus posing a threat to both animal and human health (Aarestrup, 1999). Consequently, the European Union has banned the use of in-feed antibiotics as growth promoters for animals since January 2006. A ban of using in-feed antibiotics was introduced in Denmark already in 2000, but the experience has been a dramatic increase in post-weaning diarrhoea and a concomitant increase in mortality, compromised welfare and deteriorated feed conversion efficiency in the period after weaning (Callesen, 2004). The consequence has been that producers therapeutically treat piglets displaying signs of diarrhoea with antibiotics. The increased use of antibiotic for therapeutic use together with the persistent occurrence of diarrhoea after weaning has increased costs. Furthermore it contributes to antibiotic resistance and has resulted in increased calls for a greater understanding of nutritional strategies for improved gut health of piglets.

One approach is the dietary manipulation of the gut environment by the use of feed additives, or by choice of dietary raw materials that may influence the luminal environment throughout the entire length of the intestinal tract and thereby improving 'gut health'. As discussed by Montagne *et al.* (2003), the concept of 'gut health' is complex and, at present, it is an ill-defined notion. Conway (1994) proposed that there are three major components of 'gut health', namely the diet, the mucosa and the commensal flora (Figure 1). The mucosa is composed of the digestive epithelium, the gut-associated lymphoid tissue (GALT) and the mucus overlying the epithelium. The GALT, commensal bacteria, mucus and host epithelial cells interact with each other forming a fragile and dynamic equilibrium within the alimentary tract that ensures

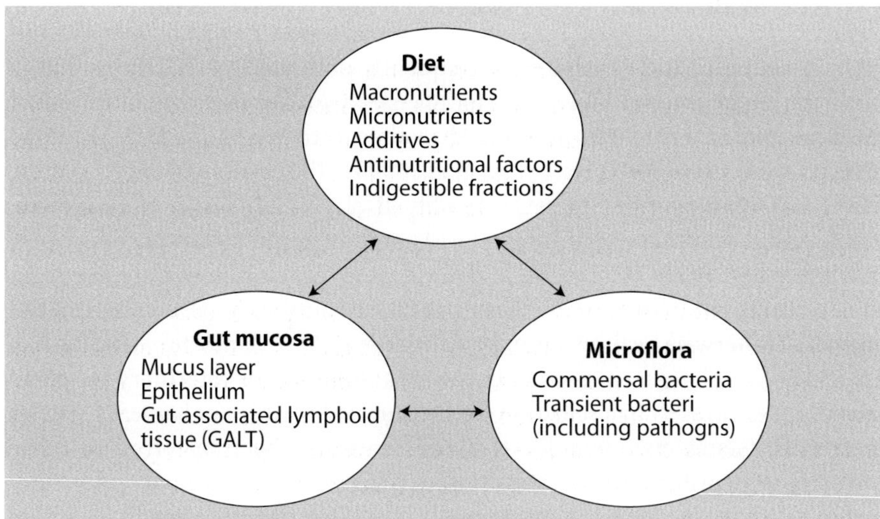

Figure 1. Schematic representation of the different elements in the gut ecosystem making up the concept of gut health. Modified from Conway (1994) as discussed by Montagne et al. *(2003).*

efficient functioning and absorption capacity of the digestive system. The feed should be selected to favour conditions in the gut that create and stabilise this balance between the host, the microflora and environment, and to prevent disturbance of the structure and function of the gut. In this respect, the relative 'gut health' value of a dietary component or diets should rest with their capacity either to stabilise or to perturb this equilibrium.

Fibre is an important component of the diet. It is resistant to digestion by endogenous enzymes in the small intestine thereby becoming the main substrate for bacterial fermentation, particularly in the large intestine of pigs and other non-ruminant animals (Bach Knudsen and Jørgensen, 2001). Because of the physical properties of fibre it interacts both with the microflora and the mucosa of all sites of the gastrointestinal tract. In this way it has an important role in the control of 'gut health'. This brief review will address different aspects of the chemical and physicochemical characteristics of fibre, how fibre influences the gut lumen, the commensal microbiota and interacts with the intestinal mucosa. Finally, there will be a brief discussion of how fibre may enhance 'gut health'.

2. Terminology and chemical structure

2.1. Terminology

Fibre is not a well-defined chemical entity, but a term that in both the human and animal nutritional literature has been defined by the methods applied for its analysis. There are numerous fibre methods applied for the analysis of fibre in feedstuffs include; the crude fibre method (Henneberg and Stohmann, 1859), the detergent methods – developed by Van Soest and co-workers (Van Soest, 1963; Van Soest and Wine, 1967; Van Soest, 1984) – for fibre rich feedstuffs and more recently the enzymatic- or non-enzymatic gravimetric AOAC (Association of Official Analytical Chemists) procedures (Prosky *et al.*, 1985) and the enzymatic-chemical Englyst (Englyst *et al.*, 1994) and Uppsala procedures (Theander *et al.*, 1994). Figure 2 addresses this issue and shows how variable fibre values reported in the animal literature may be dependent on the methods used for its analysis. In the human nutrition literature there has been a continuous debate for more than a quarter of a century concerning the definition of fibre (dietary), but no universal definition has yet been reached (Gray, 2006). For the purpose of this paper the term fibre will be restricted to the sum of non-starch polysaccharides (NSP) plus lignin, but we will also discuss dietary carbohydrate components that have similar physiological/

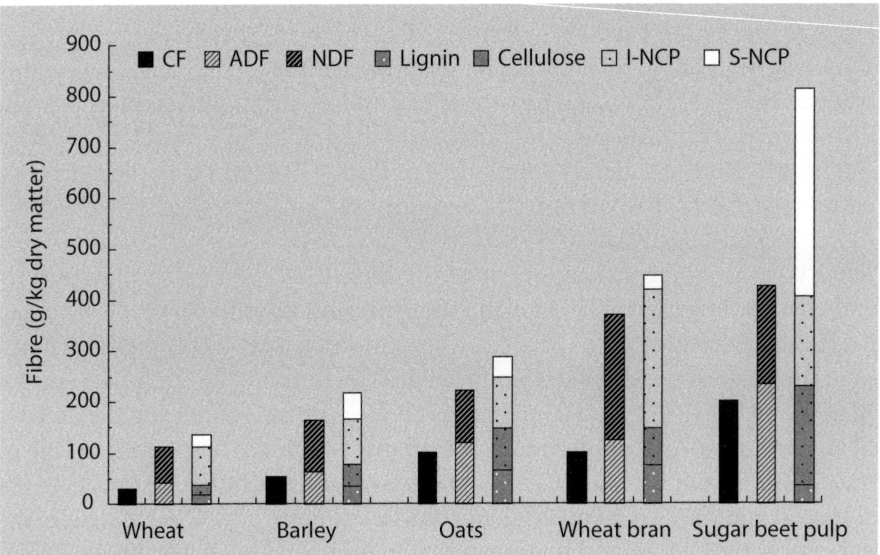

Figure 2. Analytical values for fibre in different feedstuffs as evaluated by the crude fibre (CF) method, the detergent acid detergent fibre (ADF) and neutral detergent fibre (NDF) methods of Van Soest and lignin (Klason), cellulose, insoluble non-cellulosic polysaccharides (I-NCP) and soluble non-cellulosic polysaccharides (S-NCP) obtained when using the enzymatic-chemical-gravimetric Uppsala and Englyst methods.

nutritional properties like fibre, i.e. resistant starch (RS) and non-digestible oligosaccharides (NDO). The major NSP's, RS's and NDO's present in feedstuffs are listed in Table 1.

2.2. Chemical structure of the plant cell wall

Fibre derives mainly from the plant cell walls, but some plants may also contain fibre as storage NSP. The plant cell wall consists of a series of polysaccharides often associated and/or substituted with proteins and phenolic compounds, in some cells together with the phenolic polymer lignin (Selvendran, 1984; Bacic *et al.*, 1988; Theander *et al.*, 1989). As shown in the cell wall model in Figure 3, the plant cell wall is a biphasic structure in which microfibrils of cellulose form a rigid skeleton, which is embedded in a gel-like matrix composed of NCP and glycoproteins (Carpita and Gibeaut, 1993; McDougall *et al.*, 1996). The cellulose microfibrils are highly ordered, whereas the amorphous region is less ordered. The building blocks of the cell wall polysaccharides are the pentoses arabinose and xylose, the hexoses glucose, galactose and mannose,

Table 1. Carbohydrates and lignin in feedstuffs and feed additives.

Category	Monomeric residues	Examples of source
Non-digestible oligosaccharides (DP 3-9)		
α-galactosides (Raffinose, stachyose, verbascose)	Galactose, glucose, fructose	Soybean meal, peas, rape seed meals etc.
Fructo-oligosaccharides	Fructose	Cereals, feed additives
Trans-galactooligosaccharides	Galactose, glucose	Feed additives
Xylo-oligosaccharides	Xylose, arabinose	Feed additives
Polysaccharides (DP≥10)		
A. Resistant starch (RS)		
Physical inaccessible - RS1	Glucose	Peas, faba beans
Native - RS2	Glucose	Potato
Retrograded - RS3	Glucose	Heat treated starch rich products
Chemically modified – RS_4	Glucose	Chemically modified starch
B. Non-starch (NSP)		
Cell Wall NSP		
Cellulose	Glucose	Most feedstuffs
Mixed linked β-glucans	Glucose	Barley, oats, rye
Arabinoxylans	Xylose, arabinose	Rye, wheat, barley, cereals by-products
Arabinogalactans	Galactose, arabinose	Cereal flours
Xyloglucans	Glucose, xylose	Pea hulls
Rhamnogalacturans	Uronic acids, rhamnose	Soybean meal, sugar beet fibre/pulp
Galactans	Galactose	Lupins
Non-cell Wall NSP		
Fructans	Fructose	Jerusalem artichoke, chicory roots, rye
Mannans	Mannose	Coconut cake, palm cake
Pectins	Uronic acids, rhamnose	Feed additives
Guar gum	Galactose, mannose	Feed additives
Lignin	Phenylpropanoid	Barley hulls, oat hulls,

DP: degree of polymerisation; RS: resistant starch; NSP: non-starch polysaccharides.

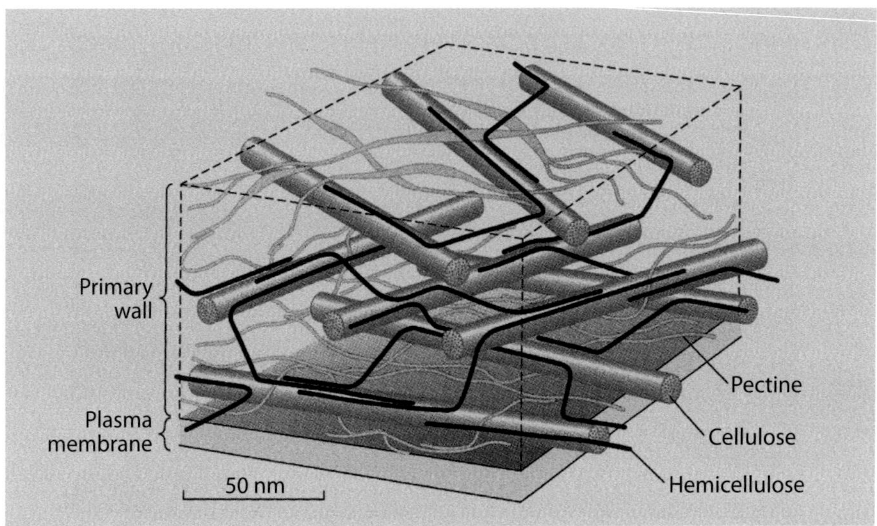

Figure 3. A three-dimensional model of the plant cell wall. McCann and Roberts (1991).

the 6-deoxyhexoses rhamnose and fucose, and the uronic acids glucuronic and galacturonic acids (or its 4-O-methyl ether). The main polysaccharides of plant cell walls are cellulose, arabinoxylans, mixed linked β(1->3)(1->4)-D-glucan (β-glucan), xyloglucans, rhamnogalacturonans, and arabinogalactans to mention the major ones (Figure 4) (Selvendran, 1984; Bacic *et al.*, 1988; Theander *et al.*, 1989). The other major component of the cell wall is lignin (Liyama *et al.*, 1994). Lignin can be described as a branched network built up by phenylpropanoid residues. In the cell wall, lignin is partly linked to non-cellulosic polysaccharides (NCP) and serves principally two main functions; it cements and anchors the cellulose microfibrils and other matrix polysaccharides, and because the lignin-polysaccharide complexes are hard, they stiffen the walls thus preventing biochemical degradation and physical damage of the walls.

The composition of the cell wall varies largely between different plant materials and plant tissues within the plant. While the nature of cellulose varies little between plants, the composition of the amorphous matrix usually shows considerable variation from tissue to tissue within the plant and between plants. In cereals, monocotyledonous plants, the main cell wall polysaccharides of whole grain cereals are arabinoxylans, cellulose, and β-glucan with some variation between the cereals (Theander *et al.*, 1989; Bach Knudsen, 1997). While cereals are virtually free of pectic substances, pectic polysaccharides are

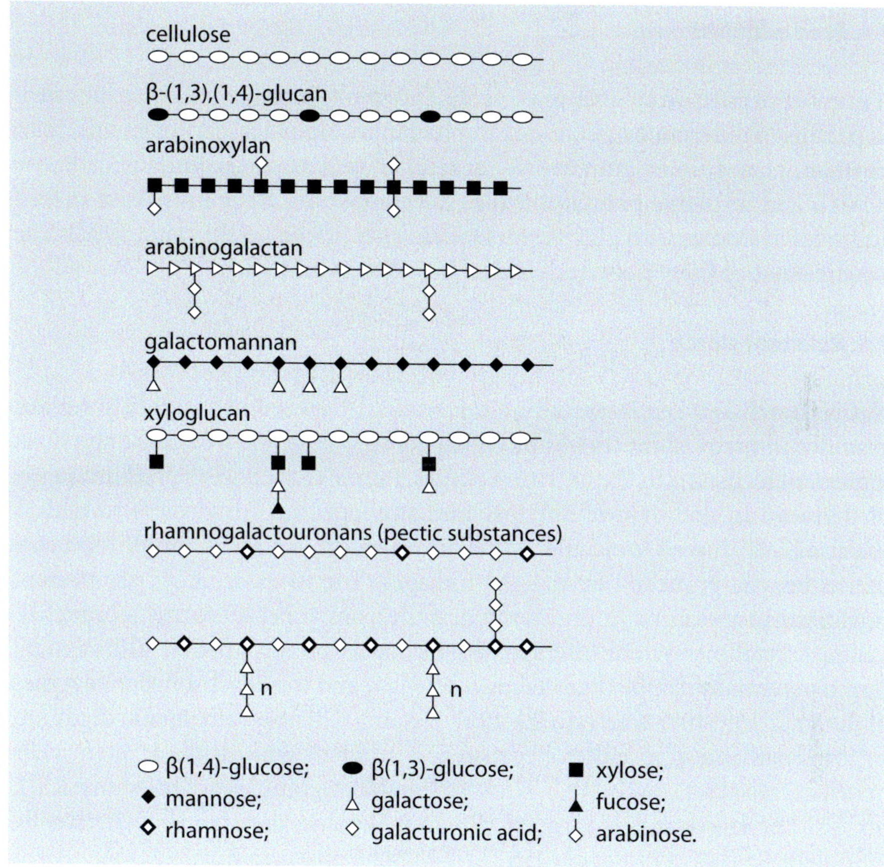

Figure 4. Schematic representation of the major cell wall polysaccharides.

found in high levels in dicotyledonous plants. Furthermore, the composition of the plant cell wall is not only dependent of the plant species in question, but also of the tissues type and the maturity of the plant organ at harvesting for feed.

2.3. Non-cell wall polysaccharides

Some plant materials also contain intracellular NSP as storage carbohydrates such as fructans in Jerusalem artichoke and chicory roots, and as mannans in palm and coconut cake. In contrast to the plant cell wall, no lignin is associated with storage NSP.

2.4. Feed additives

A number of purified soluble and viscous and non-viscous polysaccharides such as pectins of different origin, for example, inulin, alginates, carrageenans, gum xanthan, guar gum or gum arabic (acacia) as well as carboxymethylcellulose (CMC) and insoluble polysaccharides as cellulose are frequently used as feed additives in studies with piglets (McDonald *et al.*, 1999; Lærke *et al.*, 2001). The practical use of these polysaccharides, however, is limited.

2.5. Resistant starch

Native starch is a semi-crystalline material synthesised as roughly spherical granules in many plant tissues of which cereals, peas and beans are the most important feedstuffs in the nutrition of pigs. Pure starch consists predominantly of α-glucan in the form of amylose and amylopectin. Amylose is roughly a linear α(1-4)- linked molecule, while amylopectin is a much larger molecule that is heavily branched by α(1-6)- linkages. The two α-glucans are present in various proportions in the starch granules; amylopectin forms a branched helical crystalline system interspersed with amorphous lamella. Although all starch potentially can be digested by α-amylase and the brush-border enzymes in the small intestine, a certain fraction of starch will resist enzymatic digestion in the small intestine either because it is trapped within whole plant cells matrices (resistant starch, RS_1), because the starch granules are resistant (RS_2), because the starch is retrograded (RS_3), or because the starch is chemically modified (RS_4) (Englyst *et al.*, 1992).

2.6. Non-digestible oligosaccharides

NDO are present naturally in a number of predominantly protein rich feedstuffs as α-galactosides – raffinose, stachyose, verbascose and ajugose or as fructooligosaccharides that are part of the fructan fraction in Jerusalem artichoke and chicory roots. NDO may also be incorporated into the pig's diet as isolates of fructooligosaccharides from partly hydrolysed inulin or enzymatically synthesised, as trans-galactooligosaccharides or as xylo-oligosaccharides to mention the major ones (Flickinger *et al.*, 2003).

The diverse carbohydrate composition of common feedstuffs used for feeding in the pig industry is shown in Table 2.

Table 2. Carbohydrate and lignin content (g/kg dry matter) of feedstuffs (Data from Bach Knudsen, 1997 and Serena and Bach Knudsen, 2007).

Feedstuff	Sugars	NDO	Starch	Fructans[1]	S-NCP[2]	I-NCP[3]	Cellulose[3]	KL[3]	Fibre
Rice	2	2	840	<1	9	1	3	8	22
Corn	17	3	690	6	9	66	22	11	108
Wheat	13	6	651	15	25	74	20	19	138
Barley	16	6	587	4	56	88	43	35	221
Oats	13	5	468	3	40	110	82	66	298
Wheat bran	37	16	222	20	29	273	72	75	449
Barley hulls	21	12	174	7	20	267	192	115	594
Peas	39	49	454	ND	52	76	53	12	192
Soybean meal	77	60	27	ND	63	92	62	16	233
Rape seed cake	72	16	15	ND	43	103	59	90	295
Potato pulp	<1	ND	249	ND	280	95	202	35	612
Sugar beet pulp	38	ND	5	0	290	27	203	37	737
Chicory roots	156	ND	ND	470	76	24	48	11	158

NDO: non-digestible oligosaccharides; S-NCP: soluble non-cellulosic polysaccharides; I-NCP: insoluble non-cellulosic polysaccharides; KL: Klason lignin; ND: not determined.

[1] Fructans are a mix of oligosaccharides (DP 3-9) and polysaccharides (DP≥10).

[2] S-NCP is synonymous with soluble fibre.

[3] The sum of I-NCP, cellulose and KL is insoluble fibre.

3. Physico-chemical properties of fibre

The physicochemical properties – hydration properties and viscosity – of fibre are linked to the type of polymers that make up the cell wall and their intermolecular association (McDougall *et al.*, 1996). The hydration properties are characterised by the swelling capacity, solubility, water holding capacity, and water binding capacity (WBC). The latter two have been used interchangeably in the literature since both reflect the ability of a fibre source to immobilise water within its matrix. The first part of the solubilisation process of polymers is swelling in which incoming water spreads the macromolecules until they are fully extended and dispersed (imagine how the cell wall in Figure 3 expands in the three dimensional space) (Thibault *et al.*, 1992). Fibre swells to a variable extent in water: for example, isolated pectin swells greatly, but when contained within the mesh of less hydrophilic substances, the swelling is restricted. Solubilisation is not possible in the case of polysaccharides that adopt regular, ordered structures (e.g. cellulose or linear arabinoxylans), where the linear structure increases the strength of the non-covalent bonds, which stabilise the ordered conformation. Under these conditions only swelling can occur (Thibault *et al.*, 1992). From Table 3 it is clear that the fibre sources with pectin containing components, i.e. pea cotyledon, potato pulp and sugar beet pulp swells and hold water to a larger extent than is the case with hulls. Since swelling and WBC, in addition to the chemical structure of the molecules and particle size, is determined by the pH and electrolyte concentration of the surrounding fluid, fibre may swell to a variable extent during passage of the gut (Canibe and Bach Knudsen, 2002).

The majority of polysaccharides give viscous solutions when dissolved in water (Morris, 1992). The viscosity is dependent on the primary structure, molecular weight of the polymer, and the concentration. Large molecules increase the viscosity of diluted solutions and their ability to do this depends primarily on the volume they occupy. The volume of the polymers is much greater than of monomers and the volume occupied by one polymer coil will be greater than the combined volume of two coils each half its length.

Table 3. Swelling and water binding capacity and fibre content of selected feedstuffs (Data from Canibe and Bach Knudsen, 2002 and Serena and Bach Knudsen, 2007).

Feedstuff	Fibre g/kg dry matter	Swelling L/kg dry matter	Water binding capacity kg/kg dry matter
Wheat	128	2.9	1.2
Barley	217	4.0	1.5
Dehulled barley	160	5.0	1.3
Barley hulls	540	6.3	2.6
Pea cotyledon	485	11.3	7.6
Pea hulls	857	6.1	3.6
Potato pulp	612	10.8	7.2
Sugar beet pulp	737	8.7	8.7

4. The action of fibre in stomach and small intestine

4.1. Physical environment

As discussed above it is not surprising that the different types of fibre will influence the gastrointestinal environment to a variable extent. Soluble fibre sources will generally increase luminal viscosity and in most cases also the WBC in the intestinal content of stomach and the small intestine. This is illustrated in Table 4, showing the results from a study with piglets fed a low fibre control diet based on wheat and barley flour, or four diets with added barley hulls and high-methylated (HM) pectin at two variable concentrations. Pectin was the primary factor influencing luminal viscosity in the contents from the two sampling sites. For WBC, the fibre level had a more significant impact in the stomach whereas pectin was the factor raising WBC in the distal small intestine (Lærke *et al.*, 2003).

The effect of fibre on the luminal environment, however, is to a large degree influenced by the type and the chemical nature of the polysaccharides. This is shown by the results with piglets fed a control wheat, barley and soybean meal diet or the same diet in which 32 g/kg of wheat was substituted with pectins with variable degrees of esterification (DE) and calcium sensitivity in Figure 5 (Lærke *et al.*, 2001). DM80 was highly methylated pectin with a DE of approximately 80%, DM60, DM46 and DM5 had DEs of approximately

Table 4. Effects of diets varying in content and proportions of soluble and insoluble fibre on gastric and distal small intestinal viscosity and water binding capacity (Data from Lærke et al.*, 2003).*

Diet	Fibre		Viscosity mPa.s		WBC kg/kg DM	
	g/kg DM	% Soluble	Stomach	Distal SI	Stomach	Distal SI
Low fibre	73	61	1.2^{b}	1.9^{b}	1.2^{b}	4.6^{ab}
Medium fibre hull	104	37	1.2^{b}	1.6^{b}	1.2^{b}	3.3^{b}
Medium fibre pectin	104	68	5.0^{a}	7.9^{a}	1.7^{a}	5.2^{a}
High fibre hull	147	31	1.2^{b}	1.9^{b}	1.9^{a}	3.3^{b}
High fibre hull + pectin	143	40	2.4^{ab}	5.7^{a}	2.1^{a}	6.7^{a}

WBC: water-binding capacity; DM :dry matter; SI: small intestine.

60, 46 and 5%, respectively. In the study were also used two pectins classified as calcium-sensitive (CAS) and calcium-insensitive (CAN) as well as pectins isolated from sugar beet pulp (SB). From Figure 5 it is clear that the same concentration of pectins introduces significant differences in luminal viscosity. The highest values were obtained for DM80 and DM60; intermediate viscosities were obtained with CAS, DM46, CAN and SB, while DM5 did not create viscosity significantly different from the control group. The variation in viscosity between the different types of pectins was largely determined by the solubility of the pectin. When the viscosity of digesta was compared with the viscosity of pure solutions at a comparable concentration it became clear that there was a dissimilar order of viscosity elevating properties seen in water and the gastrointestinal content. Thus, although the viscosity of pure solutions of DM60, DM46 and DM5 at the same concentration was almost identical, decreasing viscosities in gut contents were seen with lower DE. This is likely due to the pectins structure and different sensitivities and reactions with components in the gastrointestinal environment.

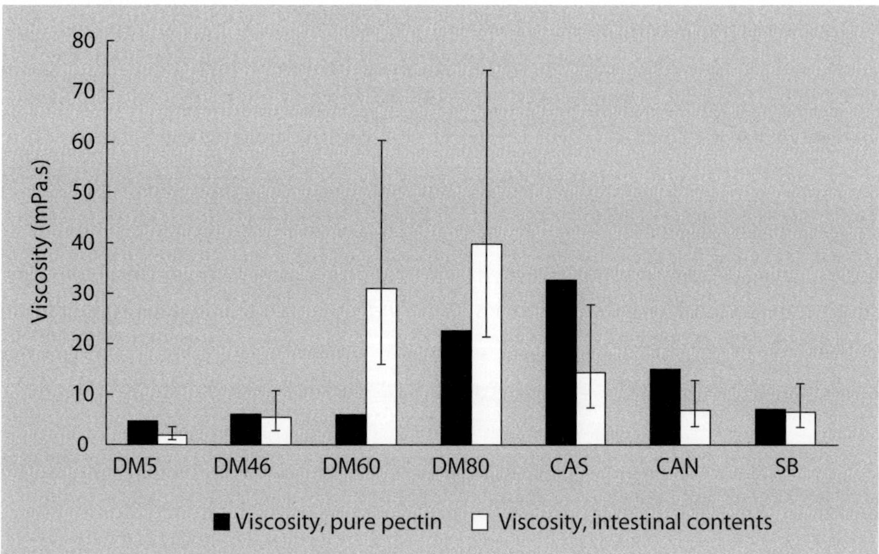

Figure 5. The viscosity of different pectins in water at a concentration of 9.6 g/L (Black bars) and in the distal thirds of the small intestine of piglets three weeks post-weaning (white bars, mean values with their 95% confidence interval, n = 8). Data from Lærke et al. *(2001).*

The intermolecular organisation and the cross-links of polysaccharides within the cell wall matrix is furthermore a factor of great importance to consider. For instance, although sugar beet pulp has a high proportion of soluble fibre (Table 2, Figures 3-4) in the form of pectin-containing components (like pectin SB; Figure 5), the viscosity-elevating properties of sugar beet pulp is much lower than anticipated from the dietary level of soluble fibre (Miquel *et al.*, 2001). On the other hand, β-glucan the major cell wall polysaccharide of barley and oat endosperm and subaleurone cell walls will to some extent solubilise from the cell wall matrix and raise luminal viscosity as demonstrated in Figure 6 (Jensen *et al.*, 1998; Hopwood *et al.*, 2004) although not nearly to the extent of what can be achieved with isolated β-glucan, pectins or other isolated fibre sources (McDonald *et al.*, 1999; Lærke *et al.*, 2001, 2003).

A factor that has significant suppressive influence on the luminal viscosity of soluble fibre is the commensal microflora. In a study by Johansen *et al.* (1997) it was found that between 25 and 55% of β-glucan in coarsely ground oat bran and between 35 and 63% of β-glucan in finely ground oat bran was solubilised in the stomach and the small intestine, but because of the significant depolymerisation of the β-glucan in the upper intestinal tract (up to 20 fold compared to the molecular weight of ingested β-glucan) there was a correspondingly lower increase in viscosity of the luminal contents as expected from the dietary concentration.

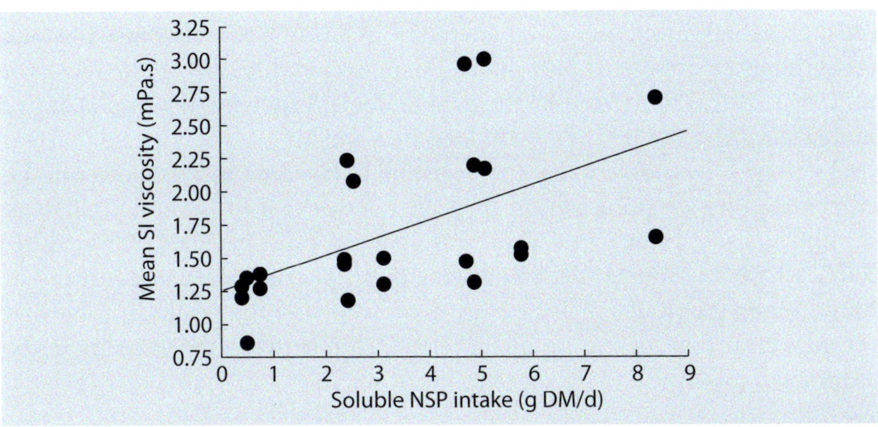

Figure 6. Relationship between the intake of soluble NSP and viscosity of pooled small intestinal content of newly weaned pigs fed a cooked rice-based diet with varying levels of pearled barley inclusion (r^2 0.298, P=0.007). SI, small intestine. Data from Hopwood et al. *(2004).*

Not only does the commensal microflora colonising the upper intestinal tract interact with the feed polysaccharides, but so will bacterial enzymes deriving from coprophagy of the piglets own faeces. This phenomenon can explain why the luminal viscosity after consuming the same β-glucan rich oat bran diet was much lower (10-20 mPas vs. ~400 mPas) when pigs were kept on concrete floor compared to housed in metabolic crates (Johansen *et al.*, 1996, 1997). The structural complexity of the NSP, however, is very important for the resistance against microbial degradation, explicitly pointed out by the higher resistance against degradation of arabinoxylans which has a far more complex chemical structure compared with β-glucan (Bach Knudsen *et al.*, 2005).

4.2. Digestion processes

Fibre will stimulate the endogenous secretions and, for some fibre, raise luminal viscosity thereby potentially interfering with the digestion processes in the small intestine by hindering the contact between the substrate and digestive enzymes and by slowing down the movements of hydrolytic products of the digestion processes. In this way fibre can reduce the uptake of glucose and delay peak blood glucose concentrations (Ellis *et al.*, 1995). However, while this may occur for diets supplemented with purified viscous polysaccharides such as guar gum (Ellis *et al.*, 1995) there is little evidence that the levels of soluble NSP present in natural feedstuffs will influence the digestion and absorption processes to any larger extent (Bach Knudsen *et al.*, 2005). A factor that is of far bigger importance in the immediate post-weaning period is the change in small intestinal morphology and alteration in enzyme activity caused among other things by a reduced feed intake (Hampson and Kidder, 1986; Pluske *et al.*, 1997). This is illustrated by the data in Table 5 showing the results of five studies covering the periods 9-28 days after weaning (piglets weaned at 3-4 weeks of age). It is evident that the digestibility of starch is much lower in the immediate post-weaning period than after 3 weeks post-weaning (Gdala *et al.*, 1997; Jensen, 1998; Lærke *et al.*, 2003; Hopwood *et al.*, 2004; Pluske *et al.*, 2007), where it is comparable to growing pigs (Bach Knudsen and Jørgensen, 2001). When the results in Table 5 are compared with the results in Table 4, it becomes clear that there is no direct relationship between the viscosity in the distal small intestine and the digestibility of starch.

4.3. Microbial activity and community

Studies performed using culture based techniques as well as molecular approaches have all confirmed the general view that the microbial community

Table 5. Digestibility of starch and non-starch polysaccharides in piglets in the post-weaning period fed diets varying in content and proportions of soluble and insoluble non-starch polysaccharides.

Diet	NSP		Starch %		NSP %	
	g/kg DM	% Soluble	Distal SI	Rectum	Distal SI	Rectum
9 days post-weaning: Lærke *et al.* (2003).						
Low fibre	65	61	83.2	99.3	36.3[a]	81.9[a]
Medium fibre hull	84	37	76.7	98.9	1.6[b]	31.4[bc]
Medium fibre pectin	86	68	75.2	97.0	2.2[b]	82.1[a]
High fibre hull	119	31	74.8	98.8	-0.2[b]	31.3[c]
High fibre hull + pectin	124	40	74.7	99.2	-24.2[b]	59.2[b]
10 days post-weaning: Hopwood *et al.* (2004).						
CR:PB 100:0	7	35	75.8	100.0		
CR:PB 75:25	26	52	66.3	99.6		
CR:PB 50:50	45	55	77.5	99.1		
CR:PB 25:97	74	49	49.0	98.4		
14 days post-weaning: Pluske *et al.* (2007).						
Medium-grain rice	~7		96.2	99.8		
Long grain rice	~7		88.6	99.8		
Waxy rice	~7		99.1	99.9		
Wheat, barley, lupins			88.5	97.6		
21 days post-weaning: Jensen *et al.* (1998).						
Covered barley	178	19	96.7	99.2	17.8	54.5
Hulless barley	142	33	94.9	99.2	30.0	76.1
28 days post-weaning: Gdala *et al.* (1997).						
Wheat, barley	166	24	98.8[a]	100	8.2	68.0
Wheat, barley, peas	173	21	95.5[b]	100	1.0	70.7

NSP: non-starch polysaccharides; SI: small intestine; CR: cooked rice; PB: pearled barley.

is very unstable in the immediate post-weaning period (Konstantinov *et al.*, 2004; Zoetendal *et al.*, 2004; Hill *et al.*, 2005; Janczyk *et al.*, 2007). It takes at least 5-10 days for the intestinal bacterial community to re-establish and to adapt its activity to the new feeding situation with complex plant materials at the expense of liquid nutrients from milk (Konstantinov *et al.*, 2004; Hill *et al.*, 2005; Janczyk *et al.*, 2007). As long as the microbial community is stable and not disturbed by enterobacteria, members of the lactobacilli family are the dominating bacterial groups and lactic acid by far the most important metabolic end-products increasing several-fold in the first 11 days after weaning and with a concomitant drop in pH (Konstantinov *et al.*, 2004; Hill *et al.*, 2005; Janczyk *et al.*, 2007). A recent study showed that there was little variation in the lactobacilli community in the immediate post-weaning period and that feeding either corn-, wheat- or barley-based diets, did not alter the lactobacilli community or the metabolic end-product composition (Hill *et al.*, 2005). The lack of response to feeding the three types of cereals is likely due to the high accumulation of residual starch in the terminal small intestine completely overshadowing the fibre effects of the three cereals. Including fructo-oligosaccharides at levels of 10 and 40 g/kg, however, increased the lactic acid concentration, reduced pH and increased the counts of Lactobacilli and Bifidobacteria (Houdijk *et al.*, 2002).

4.4. Gut morphology

The morphology of the small intestine of piglets undergoes rapid and dramatic changes at weaning; the villi shorten considerably and the crypts deepen (Hampson and Kidder, 1986). It is widely established that the post-weaning feed intake is of outmost importance for the digestive development of pigs and several authors have found that the effect of diet composition on mucosal integrity in the small intestine was overridden by diminished feed intake (van Beers-Schreurs *et al.*, 1998; Spreeuwenberg *et al.*, 2001).

The addition of soluble fibre to the diet of piglets generally causes an increase in the viscosity of the intestinal content (Table 4, Figure 5), which may increase the rate of villus cell losses leading to villus atrophy. This has been seen in studies using pectin (Hedemann *et al.*, 2006) and CMC (a water soluble synthetic viscous polysaccharide which is resistant to microbial fermentation; McDonald *et al.*, 2001). However, in the study of McDonald *et al.* (2001) pigs fed a low-viscosity CMC had increased villus height suggesting that viscosity may be beneficial up to a threshold. Using CMC in piglet feed increased the crypt depth (McDonald *et al.*, 2001) whereas pectin-fed piglets had lower crypts than piglets fed a low fibre diet (Hedemann *et al.*, 2006) suggesting that the type of soluble fibre influences the response. The villus height/crypt depth ratio is a useful criterion for estimating the likely digestive capacity of the small intestine. When feeding high-viscosity CMC the ratio decreased (McDonald *et al.*, 2001) whereas it was maintained when feeding pectin (Hedemann *et al.*, 2006).

Inclusion of 10% wheat straw, insoluble fibre, to a low fibre diet resulted in deeper crypts in the jejunum and ileum and augmented cell division in growing pigs (Jin *et al.*, 1994). Similar results were not found in newly-weaned piglets where fibre concentration (7.3 vs. 14.5% of DM) did not affect the intestinal morphology (Hedemann *et al.*, 2006). The increased crypt-cell proliferation induced by fibre may be explained by the trophic effect of short-chain fatty acids (SCFA) and especially butyrate. The effect of SCFA is not restricted to the colon, and SCFA also stimulate cell proliferation and growth of the small intestine. In piglets the microflora may, however, not be fully adapted to fibre (Jensen, 1998).

5. The action of fibre in large intestine

5.1. Fermentation and fermentation end-products

The low digestibility of starch in the small intestine will have a major impact on the composition of the digesta solids available for fermentation during the first two-weeks post-weaning; thereafter digesta solids will be largely determined by fibre content and composition (Bach Knudsen, 2001a). The high load of starch to the large intestine the first two weeks after weaning, however, does not seem to have a major influence on the fibre degradation as indicated by the rectal digestibility of NSP in Table 5. The likely cause is that the hydrolytic capacity of the microflora in the large intestine is more than sufficient for efficient degradation of all but the most difficult degradable fibre components. This was also the conclusion drawn by Longland *et al.* (1994) and is illustrated by the results in Figure 7 showing the increasing digestibility of NSP residues from the ileum to faeces of piglets that were fed a diet consisting of cereals and soybean meal as sole plant components (Gdala *et al.*, 1997). Based on the composition of the plant materials, galactose and uronic acids can be regarded as markers for pectin-containing materials deriving predominantly from soybean meal, xylose as a marker for arabinoxylans from cereals and glucose as a marker of β-glucan and cellulose. Thus, pectin-containing materials and β-glucan are primarily

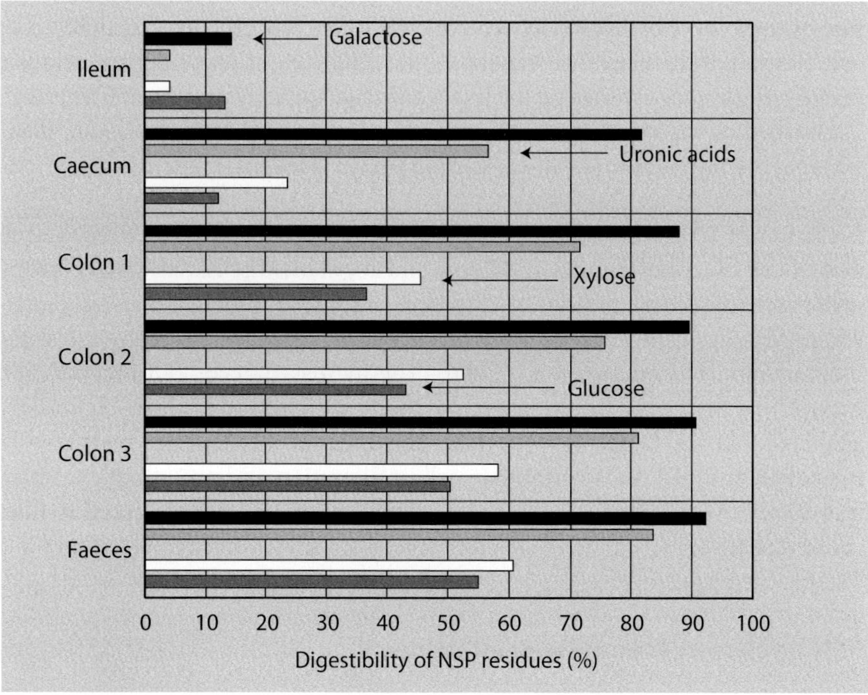

Figure 7. Digestibility of non-starch polysaccharide residues from ileum to faeces of piglets fed a cereal-soybean meal as sole plant materials. Data from Gdala et al. *(1997).*

digested in the caecum and the proximal part of the colon, arabinoxylans up to the middle part of the colon while cellulose is digested at the more distal part of colon. The mean transit time in the caecum and colon was estimated to be 2.6 h and 18.1 h, respectively. Similar results were found when piglets were fed naked and covered barley where more than 95% of β-glucan had been degraded in the caecum (Jensen *et al.*, 1998).

The concentration of SCFA in the colon content is increased post-weaning (van Beers-Schreurs *et al.*, 1998; Bruininx *et al.*, 2004), and although the concentration of SCFA in the lumen of the large intestine in piglets is comparable to what is found with older animals (growing pigs and sows) the type of substrate may have a profound influence on the composition of fermentation end-products. For instance, inclusion of RS_2 from raw potato in diets for piglets stimulated butyrate formation (Table 6; Hedemann and Bach Knudsen, 2007). The same was the case when the wheat, barley and lupins diet with low pre-caecal

Table 6. Concentration and molar proportion of butyrate after consumption of diets providing various levels of starch for fermentation in the large intestine (Data from Hedemann and Bach Knudsen, 2007 and Pluske et al.*, 2007).*

	Total SCFA			Butyrate, %		
	Ce	PC	DC	Ce	PC	DC
mM						
Medium-grain rice	140[a]	121[a]	103	11[a]	13[a]	15[a]
Long grain rice	175[ab]	137[a]	110	12[a]	13[a]	15[a]
Waxy rice	145[a]	136[a]	96	11[a]	13[a]	17[a]
Wheat, barley, lupins	196[b]	213[a]	150	26[b]	25[b]	22[b]
mmol/kg						
Control	97	69	58	8	10	10
Potato starch 80	101	90	75	11	12	12
Potato starch 160	111	98	84	17	17	15
P-value						
Diet	0.0001			0.0001		
Segment	0.0001			0.64		

SCFA: short chain fatty acids; Ce: caecum; PC: proximal colon; SC: distal colon.

digestibility of starch was fed (Table 5; Pluske *et al.*, 2007). Moreover, there are findings suggesting that changes in and variation between piglets in fermentative capacity immediately after weaning is reflected not only in the concentration of SCFA, but also in fermentative profile even when diets not specifically stimulating butyrate production are used (Figure 8; Lærke *et al.*, 2007). This indicates a change and individual variation in the microbial population after weaning not specifically related to dietary composition (Jensen, 1998). From approximately 2 weeks post-feeding and onwards, the fibre polysaccharides are the main dietary factors influencing the end-product formation. Current knowledge indicate that cellulose stimulate acetate formation whereas cereals arabinoxylans stimulate butyrate formation (Bach Knudsen, 2005).

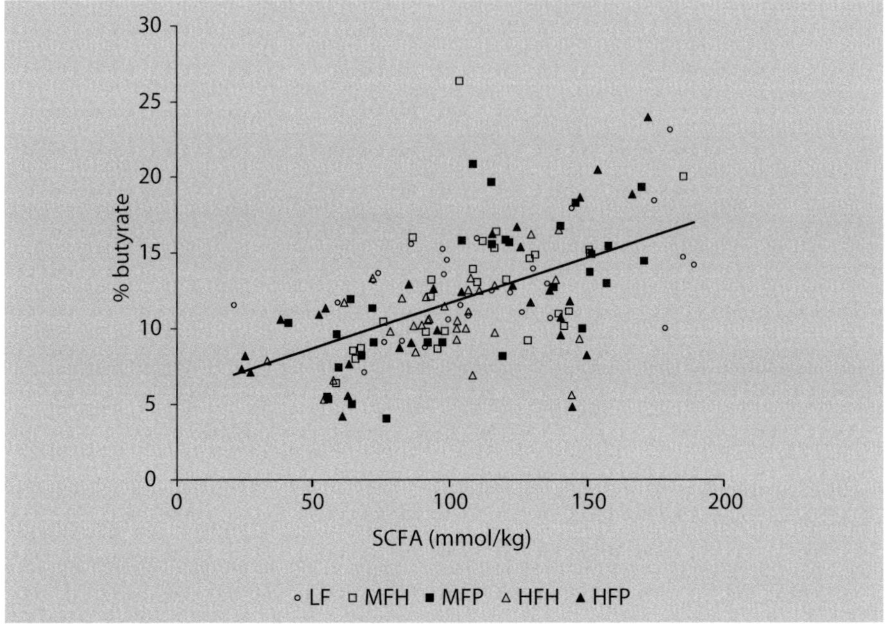

Figure 8. Relationship between the proportion of butyrate and total SCFA concentration (mmol/kg) across segments of piglets fed a low fibre diet (LF), medium fibre with the addition of barley hulls (MFH) or pectin (MFP) or high-fibre diets based on barley hulls (HFH) or a combination of barley hulls and pectin (HFP) for 9 days after weaning. Each point represents one sample (from caecum, mid, or distal colon) from one pig. The regression line is indicated as % butyrate = 0.06 x concentration of SCFA + 5.66, r^2=0.31, p=0.0001. Data from Lærke et al. *(2007).*

5.2. Physical effects

The carbohydrates will have different physical effects depending on the fat in the large intestine. The effect of extensively fermented fibre are primarily related to end products (e.g. SCFA), pH reduction and production of microbial biomass resulting in a low increase in faecal dry weight (approximately 0.3 g solid per gram fermentable carbohydrates), whereas the effects of poorly-fermented fibre depend on the physical properties (WBC) of the non-digested residue and the overall digestibility of the fibre polysaccharides. With the latter types of fibre, the increase in faecal dry weight with for example, hull will be approximately 1 g solid per gram extra NSP consumed. Since the weight of the gut content will increase in response to fermentable as well as non-fermentable carbohydrates and the gut only can expand to a certain level, and undigested residues have a stimulatory influence on the gut motility, the transit time through colon will be reduced (Bach Knudsen, 2001b).

5.3. Microbial activity and community

Long retention time, temperature, moisture content and the relatively high nutrient density are all conditions that favour a prolific growth of microorganisms, which is present at levels of 10^{10}-10^{11} culturable microorganisms per gram digesta (Jensen, 2001). In response to increased levels of fermentable carbohydrates entering the large intestine, there will be a general rise in the activity of the entire microbial community (Bach Knudsen *et al.*, 1991; Jensen and Jørgensen, 1994), but because the composition of fibre polysaccharides are complex (Figure 3-4) and require different enzymes to be hydrolysed, specific groups of microorganisms will seldom be stimulated. Fructose containing oligo- and polysaccharides, however, may specifically stimulate lactic acid bacteria (*Lactobacillus* spp. together with *Bifidobacterium* spp.) (Gibson and Wang, 1994; Gibson *et al.*, 1995; Flickinger *et al.*, 2003; Macfarlane *et al.* 2006). It is a generally held belief that stimulation of lactic acid bacteria is beneficial as attachment of these harmless bacteria to the mucosa may protect the animals from gut infection. Since inulin and fructans are readily fermentable they further, depending on the dose, reduce luminal pH (Houdijk *et al.*, 2002; Bach Knudsen *et al.*, 2003) and in this way reduce the risk of establishment of enteropathogenic strains of *Escherichia coli, Salmonella, Shingella* or some clostridia, all being pH sensitive (Gibson and Wang, 1994; Macfarlane *et al. 2006*). When growing pigs were fed a diet containing fermentable carbohydrates from chicory roots and sweet lupins and experimentally infected with *Brachyspira hyodysenteriae,* the animals were completely protected against the development of swine dysentery (Thomsen *et al.*, 2007). Terminal restriction fragment length polymorphism analysis of colonic content suggest that pigs fed the fructan-rich chicory root diet had a higher proportion of *Bifidobacterium thermoacidophilum* and *Megasphaera elsdenii*, which inhibited *B. hyodysenteriae* to be established (Mølbak *et al.*, 2007). An improved ratio between lactobacilli and coliform and reduced luminal pH in digesta have also been found in a study with piglets fed diets containing inulin (Wellock *et al.*, 2007).

5.4. Gut morphology

Studies on the morphological development of the large intestine in piglets are scarce. A recent study has shown that the crypt depth increased during the first 5 days post-weaning (Hedemann *et al.*, 2007). The main energy source for the colonic epithelium is SCFA and preferentially butyrate (Scheppach, 1994). The concentration of SCFA in the colon content is increased post-weaning (van Beers-Schreurs *et al.*, 1998; Bruininx *et al.*, 2004) and hence energy is available for the growth of the colonic epithelium. In a study where piglets were fed pectin and barley hulls as fibre sources for 9 days post-weaning we found that piglets fed pectin had the lowest crypts (Hedemann *et al.*, 2006). The differences in crypt depth could not be attributed to differences in SCFA concentration in colonic material as no differences in SCFA concentration due to dietary treatments were observed (unpublished results). Whether feed intake influences the morphology of the large intestine is unknown, however the feed intake of the pectin-fed piglets was lower than that of piglets fed barley hulls. In another study, feeding diets differing in content and composition of fibre for 2 weeks post-weaning did not induce any differences in colonic morphology (Piel *et al.*, 2007) in spite of large differences in fibre content (134 vs. 217 g/kg DM). In the literature, the effect of fibre on colonic morphology is conflicting concerning growing pigs as well. It depends on the botanic origin and fermentation properties of the fibre and the composition of the microflora in the colon of pigs (Williams *et al.*, 2001). During the first two weeks after weaning, the contribution of starch as fermentable carbohydrates for fermentation in the large intestine (Table 5) can easily out-weigh fibre and therefore the effects of fibre on the concentration and composition of SCFA may be minor, resulting in no or minimal effects on intestinal morphology.

Another mechanism by which the fibre can be involved in the protection of pathogenic diseases is by the stimulation that the lactic acid bacteria may have on the immune system. Lactobacilli interact with the immune cells in the GALT, modifying the proportion of T-cells (CD4+ and CD8) and B-cells, macrophages, production of anti- and proinflammatory cytokines, and immunoglobilins, particularly IgA. The influence on the immune system is thought to be both through immediate contact of bacteria with immune cells and via the production of SCFA which can stimulate immune lymphocytes (Schley and Field, 2002; Macfarlane *et al.* 2006). A more direct effect of fibre is through the direct stimulation of the mucin production in the gut (Schley and Field, 2002; Montagne *et al.*, 2003).

6. Fibre and feed intake and performance

The direct effect of fibre on VFI and performance in the immediate post-weaning period is not easy to quantify because of the huge variability in VFI and performance during the first 2-3 weeks after feeding. However, soluble viscous fibre such as some types of pectins and guar gum seem consistency to reduce VFI and performance, whereas total and insoluble fibre up to a certain level are of less importance (Longland *et al.*, 1994; McDonald *et al.*, 1999; Pedersen *et al.*, 2003). The high variability in VFI and performance also makes it difficult to establish relationships between events in the gastrointestinal tract and these parameters. For instance, in a recent study involving rice with different characteristics and a wheat, barley, and lupin diet it was not possible to identify any significant relationship between the variation in the ileal digestibility of starch and the performance post-weaning (Pluske *et al.*, 2007). However, a higher carcass weight percentage was seen with the rice diets compared with the more fibre-rich wheat, barley, and lupin diets.

7. Fibre and gut health

An essential question is to what extent it is possible to select either feedstuffs naturally rich in fibre or from fibre isolates that create and stabilise the balance between the host, the microflora and environment, thereby avoiding the outbreak of diarrhoea due to proliferation of enterotoxigenic bacteria? As has been discussed above, fibres are an important component of all, but a few feedstuffs (i.e. rice) used in the feeding of piglets. Fibres have numerous physicochemical properties in all segments of the gut brought about by the chemical and structural organisation of primarily the plant cell wall or fibre isolates (Figure 3 and 4). The fibre in itself will have a stabilising influence on the luminal environment by immobilising a certain fraction of the liquids, but there is a continuous debate as to whether fibre exerts beneficial or detrimental influence on the development of post-weaning enteric disorders (PWED). For example, fibre from the outer hull of barley, rich in insoluble fibre (Table 2), reduces severity of PWED (Smith and Halls, 1968) whereas feeding barley meal, which contains the soluble β-glucan has been associated with increased susceptibility to develop PWED (Smith and Halls, 1968; Hopwood *et al.*, 2004). Studies with soluble and viscous NSP in the form of guar gum and CMC have further been shown to exacerbate experimental PWED whereas an almost fibre-free cooked rice based diet was more protective (McDonald *et al.*, 1999, 2001; Montagne *et al.*, 2004). When pectins were included in either a diet based on wheat and barley flour or wholegrain wheat and barley there was no difference in the frequency of spontaneous PWED. The interaction between soluble fibre, insoluble fibre and starch on one side and the microbial community and intestinal structure and function (Figure 1) on the other side are therefore very complex and obviously require further elucidation. Although we have come a long way in obtaining analytical details of the carbohydrate fraction of feedstuffs as well as of other nutrients compared to what was possible to achieve with the classical Weende analyses, the methods we apply in nutritional and physiological research are still very crude compared to what may be needed for an in-dept understanding of how carbohydrates act and interact with the microbiota and intestine. It is obvious from the compilation above that the digestibility of starch (Table 5), and likely other macronutrients is compromised during the two first weeks after weaning, which inevitably makes interpretation of the specific fibre effects difficult. It is also obvious that a thorough investigation of the potential in using fructose containing oligo- and polymers as a means of stimulating lactic acid bacteria thereby protecting the gut against the establishment of enteropathogenic bacteria strains needs further exploitation.

8. Conclusions

The fibre fraction represents a diverse group of polymers present as cell wall and storage components in most feedstuffs. When ingested, the fibre components may interact with the digestive processes along the entire gastrointestinal tract, with the microbial community as well as with the structure and function of the gut. However, the direct effects of fibre in the first two weeks after weaning (weaning age 3-4 weeks) are blurred by an extremely variable feed intake and by the low pre-caecal starch digestibility, which makes it difficult to judge the specific effects of soluble and insoluble fibre on 'gut health'. However, a diet containing a mix of soluble and insoluble fibre and carbohydrate components that specifically stimulate lactobacilli bacteria over enteropathogenic bacteria could prove to be beneficial.

References

Aarestrup, F.M. (1999). Association between the consumption of antimicrobial agents in animal husbandry and the co-occurrence of resistance bacteria among food animals. *International Journal of Antimicrobial Agents* **12:** 279-285

Armstrong, D.G. (1986). Gut-active growth promoters. *In:* Control and Metabolism of Animal Growth, (Ed. E.A. Budding) pp. 21-37.

Bach Knudsen, K.E. (1997). Carbohydrate and lignin contents of plant materials used in animal feeding. *Animal Feed Science and Technology* **67:** 319-338.

Bach Knudsen, K.E. (2001a). Development of antibiotic resistance and options to replace antimicrobials in animal diets. *Proceedings of the Nutrition Society* **60:** 291-299.

Bach Knudsen, K.E. (2001b). The nutritional significance of "dietary fibre" analysis. *Animal Feed Science and Technology* **90:** 3-20.

Bach Knudsen, K.E. (2005). Effect of dietary non-digestible carbohydrates on the rate of SCFA delivery to peripheral tissues. *Foods & Food Ingredients Journal of Japan* **211:** 1008-1017.

Bach Knudsen, K.E., Jensen, B.B., Andersen, J.O. and Hansen, I. (1991). Gastrointestinal implications in pigs of wheat and oat fractions 2. Microbial activity in the gastrointestinal tract. *British Journal of Nutrition* **65:** 233-248.

Bach Knudsen, K.E. and Jørgensen, H. (2001). Intestinal degradation of dietary carbohydrates - from birth to maturity. *In:* Digestive Physiology of Pigs. (Eds. J.E. Lindberg and B. Ogle). CABI Publishing: Wallingford, UK. pp. 109-120.

Bach Knudsen, K.E., Petkevicius, S., Jørgensen, H. and Murrel, K.D. (2003). A high load of rapidly fermentable carbohydrates reduces worm burden in infected pigs. *In:* Manipulating pig production IX. (Ed. J.E. Paterson). Australasian Pig Science Association Inc., Werribee, Australia: pp. 169.

Bach Knudsen, K.E., Serena, A., Kjaer, A.K., Jorgensen, H. and Engberg, R. (2005). Rye bread enhances the production and plasma concentration of butyrate but not the plasma concentrations of glucose and insulin in pigs. *Journal of Nutrition* **135:** 1696-1704.

Bacic, A., Harris, P.J. and Stone, B.A. (1988). Structure and function of plant cell walls. *The Biochemistry of Plants* **14:** 297-371.

Bruininx, E.M.A.M., Schellingerhout, A.B., Binnendijk, G.P., van de Peet-Schwering, C.M.C., Schrama, J.W., Hartog, L.A., Everts, H. and Beynen, A.C. (2004). Individually assessed creep food consumption by suckled piglets: influence on post-weaning food intake characteristics and indicators of gut structure and hind-gut fermentation. *Animal Science* **78:** 67-75.

Callesen, J. (2004). Effects of termination of AGP-use on pig welfare and productivity. *In:* Beyond Antimicrobial Growth Promoters in Food Animal Production. (Eds. J.T. Sørensen and B.B. Jensen). Foulum: Danish Institute of Agricultural Sciences. pp. 57-60.

Canibe, N. and Bach Knudsen, K. (2002). Degradation and physicochemical changes of barley and pea fibre along the gastrointestinal tract of pigs. *Journal of the Science of Food and Agriculture* **82:** 27-39.

Carpita, N.C. and Gibeaut, D.M. (1993). Structural models of primary cell walls in flowering plants: Consistency of molecular structure with the physical properties of the walls during growth. *The Plant Journal* **3:** 1-30.

Conway, P. (1994). Function and regulation of the gastrointestinal microbiota of the pig. *Proceedings of the VIth International Symposium on Digestive Physiology in Pigs*, pp. 231-240.

Ellis, P.R., Roberts, F.G., Low, A.G. and Morgan, L.M. (1995). The effect of high-molecular-weight guar gum on net apparent glucose absorption and net apparent insulin and gastric inhibitory polypeptide production in the growing pig: relationship to rheological changes in jejunal digesta. *British Journal of Nutrition* **74:** 539-556.

Englyst, H.N., Kingman, S.M. and Cummings, J.H. (1992). Classification and measurement of nutritionally important starch fractions. *European Journal of Clinical Nutrition* **46**: S33-50.

Englyst, H.N., Quigley, M.E. and Hudson, G.J. (1994). Determination of dietary fibre as non-starch polysaccherides with gas-liquid chromatography, high-performance liquid chromatography or spectrophotometric measurements of constituent sugars. *Analyst* **119:** 1497-1509.

Flickinger, E.A., Van Loo, J. and Fahey, G.C. Jr. (2003). Nutritional responses to the presence of inulin and oligofructose in the diets of domesticated animals: a review. *Critical Review of Food Science and Nutrition* **43:** 19-60.

Gdala, J., Johansen, H.N., Bach Knudsen, K.E., Knap, I.H., Wagner, P. and Jorgensen, O.B. (1997). The digestibility of carbohydrates, protein and fat in the small and large intestine of piglets fed non-supplemented and enzyme supplemented diets. *Animal Feed Science and Technology* **65:** 15-33.

Gibson, G.R., Beatty, E.R., Wang, X. and Cummings, J.H. (1995). Selective Stimulation of Bifidobacteria in the Human Colon by Oligofructose and Inulin. *Gastroenterology* **108:** 975-982.

Gibson, G.R. and Wang, X. (1994). Regulatory effects of bifidobacteria on the growth of other colonic bacteria. *Journal of Applied Bacteriology* **77:** 412-420.

Gray, J. (2006). Dietary fibre: Definition, Analysis, Physiology and Health. Brussels: ILSI Europe.

Hampson, D.J., Pethick, D.W. and Pluske, J.R. (1999). Can diet be used as an alternative to antibiotics to help control enteric bacterial infections of pigs? *In:* Manipulating pig production VII. Antibiotics in pig production. Nottingham University Press, Nottingham, UK. pp. 210-219.

Hampson, J. and Kidder, D.E. (1986). Influence of creep feeding and weaning on brush border enzyme activities in the piglet small intestine. *Research in Veterinary Science* **40:** 24-31.

Hedemann, M.S. and Bach Knudsen, K.E. (2007). Resistant starch for weaning pigs - Effect on concentration of short chain fatty acids in digesta and intestinal morphology. *Livestock Science* **108:** 175-177.

Hedemann, M.S., Dybkjaer, L. and Jensen, B.B. (2007). Pre-weaning eating activity and morphological parameters in the small and large intestine of piglets. *Livestock Science* **108:** 128-131.

Hedemann, M.S., Eskildsen, M., Laerke, H.N., Pedersen, C., Lindberg, J.E., Laurinen, P. and Bach Knudsen, K.E. (2006). Intestinal morphology and enzymatic activity in newly weaned pigs fed contrasting fiber concentrations and fiber properties. *Journal of Animal Science* **84:** 1375.

Henneberg, W. and Stohmann, F. (1859) Über das Erhaltungsfutter volljährigen Rindviehs. *Journal Landwirtschaft* **3:** 485-551.

Hill, J.E., Hemmingsen, S.M., Goldade, B.G., Dumonceaux, T.J., Klassen, J., Zijlstra, R.T., Goh, S.H. and Van Kessel, A.G. (2005). Comparison of ileum microflora of pigs fed corn-, wheat-, or barley-based diets by chaperonin-60 sequencing and quantitative PCR. *Applied Environmental Microbiology* **71:** 867-875.

Hopwood, D.E., Pethick, D.W., Pluske, J.R. and Hampson, D.J. (2004). Addition of pearl barley to a rice-based diet for newly weaned piglets increases the viscosity of the intestinal contents, reduces starch digestibility and exacerbates post-weaning colibacillosis. *British Journal of Nutrition* **92:** 419-427.

Houdijk, J.G., Hartemink, R., Verstegen, M.W. and Bosch, M.W. (2002). Effects of dietary non-digestible oligosaccharides on microbial characteristics of ileal chyme and faeces in weaner pigs. *Archives of Animal Nutrition* **56:** 297-307.

Janczyk, P., Pieper, R., Smidt, H. and Souffrant, W.B. (2007). Changes in the diversity of pig ileal lactobacilli around weaning determined by means of 16S rRNA gene amplification and denaturing gradient gel electrophoresis. *FEMS Microbiology and Ecology* **61:** 132-140.

Jensen, B.B. (1998). The impact of feed additives on the microbial ecology of the gut in young pigs. *Journal of Animal and Feed Sciences* **7:** 45-64.

Jensen, B.B. (2001). Possible ways of modifying type and amount of products from microbial fermentation in the gut. *In:* Gut Environment of pigs. (Eds. A. Piva, K.E. Bach Knudsen and J.E, Lindberg). Nottingham University Press, Nottingham, UK. pp. 181-200.

Jensen, B.B. and Jørgensen, H. (1994) Effect of dietary fiber on microbial activity and microbial gas production in various regions of the gastrointestinal tract of pigs. *Applied and Environmental Microbiology* **60:** 1897-1904.

Jensen, M.S., Bach Knudsen, K.E., Inborr, J. and Jakobsen, K. (1998). Effect of [beta]-glucanase supplementation on pancreatic enzyme activity and nutrient digestibility in piglets fed diets based on hulled and hulless barley varieties. *Animal Feed Science and Technology* **72:** 329-345.

Jin, L., Reynolds, L.P., Redmer, D.A., Caton, J.S. and Crenshaw, J.D. (1994). Effects of dietary fiber on intestinal growth, cell proliferation, and morphology in growing pigs. *Journal of Animal Science* **72:** 2270-2278.

Johansen, H.N., Bach Knudsen, K.E. and Sandström, B. (1996). Effect of varying content of soluble dietary fibre from wheat flour and oat milling fractions on gastric emptying in pigs. *British Journal of Nutrition* **75:** 339-351.

Johansen, H.N., Bach Knudsen, K.E., Wood, P.J. and Fulcher, R.G. (1997). Physico-chemical properties and the digestibility of polysaccharides from oats in the gastrointestinal tract of pigs. *Journal of Science of Food and Agriculture* **73:** 81-92.

Konstantinov, S.R., Awati, A., Smidt, H., Williams, B.A., Akkermans, A.D. and de Vos, W.M. (2004). Specific response of a novel and abundant Lactobacillus amylovorus-like phylotype to dietary prebiotics in the guts of weaning piglets. *Applied and Environmental Microbiology* **70:** 3821-3830.

Liyama, K., Lam, T.B-T. and Stone, B.A. (1994). Covalent cross-linkes in the cell wall. *Plant Physiology.* **104:** 315-320.

Longland, A.C., Curruthers, J. and Low, A.G. (1994). The ability of piglets 4 to 8 weeks old to digest and perform on diets containing two contrasting sources of non-starch polysaccharides. *Animal Production* **58:** 405-419.

Lærke, H.N., Hedemann, M.S., Bach Knudsen, K.E., Laurinen, P., Lindberg, J.E. and Pedersen, C. (2007). Association between butyrate and short-chain fatty acid concentrations in gut contents and faeces in weaning piglets. *Livestock Science* **108:** 163-166.

Lærke, H.N., Hedemann, M.S., Pedersen, C., Laurinen, P., Lindberg, J.E. and Bach Knudsen, K.E. (2003). Limitation in starch digestion in the newly weaned pig. Does it relate to physico-chemical properties or enzyme activity in the gut? *In:* Proceedings of the 9th Symposium of Digestive Physiology of Pigs Vol 2. (Ed. R.O. Ball). University of Alberta, Alberta, Canada. pp. 149-151.

Lærke, H.N., Hellwing, A.L.F., Bach Knudsen, K.E., Strarup, A. and Rolin, C. (2001). Isolated pectins vary in their functional properties in the gut of piglets. *In:* Digestive Physiology of Pigs (Eds. J.E. Lindberg and B. Ogle). CABI Publishing, Wallingford, UK. pp. 127-129.

Macfarlane, S., Macfarlane, G.T. and Cummings, J.H. (2006). Review article: prebiotics in the gastrointestinal tract. *Alimentary Pharmacology and Therapeutics* **24:** 701-714.

McCann, M.C. and Roberts, K. (1991). Architecture of the primary cell wall. *In:* The Cytoskeletal Basis of Plant Growth and Form (Ed. C.W. Lloyd). Academic Press, London, pp. 109-129.

McDonald, D.E., Pethick, D.W., Mullan, B.P. and Hampson, D.J. (2001). Increasing viscosity of the intestinal contents alters small intestinal structure and intestinal growth, and stimulates proliferation of enterotoxigenic *Escherichia coli* in newly-weaned pigs. *British Journal of Nutrition* **86:** 487-498.

McDonald, D.E., Pethick, D.W., Pluske, J.R. and Hampson, D.J. (1999). Adverse effects of soluble non-starch polysaccharide (guar gum) on piglet growth and experimental colibacillosis immediately after weaning. *Research in Veterinary Science* **67:** 245-250.

McDougall, G.J., Morrison, I.M., Stewart, D. and Hillman, J.R. (1996). Plant cell walls as dietary fibre: Range, structure, processing and function. *Journal of the Science of Food and Agriculture* **70:** 133-150.

Miquel, N., Bach Knudsen, K.E. and Jørgensen, H. (2001). Impact of diets varying in dietary fibre characteristics on gastric emptying in pregnant sows. *Archives of Animal Nutrition* **55:** 121-145.

Montagne, L., Cavaney, F.S., Hampson, D.J., Lalles, J.P. and Pluske, J.R. (2004). Effect of diet composition on postweaning colibacillosis in piglets. *Journal Animal Science* **82:** 2364-2374.

Montagne, L., Pluske, J.R. and Hampson, D.J. (2003). A review of interactions between dietary fibre and the intestinal mucosa, and their consequences on digestive health in young non-ruminant animals. *Animal Feed Science and Technology* **108:**95-117.

Morris, E.R. (1992). Physico-chemical properties of food polysaccharides. *In:* Dietary fibre: A component of food: Nutritional function in health and disease. (Eds. T.F. Schweizer and C.A. Edwards). Springer-Verlag, London, pp. 41-55.

Mølbak, L., Thomsen, L., Jensen, T., Bach Knudsen, K.E. and Boye, M. (2007). Increased amount of *Bifidobacterium thermoacidophilum* and *Megashpaera elsdenii* in the colonic microbiota of pigs fed a swine dysentery preventive diet containing chicory roots and sweet lupine. *Journal of Applied Microbiology* **103**:1853-1867.

Pedersen, C., Lærke, H.N., Lindberg, J.E., Hedemann, M.S., Laurinen, P. and Bach Knudsen, K.E. (2003). Digestibility and performance in newly weaned piglets fed diets with contrasting fibre levels and fibre properties. *In:* Proceedings of the 9th Symposium of Digestive Physiology of Pigs Vol 2 (Ed. R. O. Ball). Banff, Alberta, Canada: University of Alberta Department of Agriculture, Food and Nutritional Science, pp. 128-130.

Piel, C., Montagne, L., Seve, B. and Lalles, J.P. (2007). Dietary fibre and indigestible protein increase ileal glycoprotein output without impacting colonic crypt goblet cells in weaned piglets. *Livestock Science* **108:** 106-108.

Pluske, J.R., Hampson, D.J. and Williams, I.H. (1997). Factors influencing the structure and function of the small intestine in the weaned pig: a review. *Livestock Production Science* **51:** 215-236.

Pluske, J.R., Montagne, L., Cavaney, F.S., Mullan, B.P., Pethick, D.W. and Hampson, D.J. (2007). Feeding different types of cooked white rice to piglets after weaning influences starch digestion, digesta and fermentation characteristics and the faecal shedding of beta-haemolytic *Escherichia coli*. *British Journal of Nutrition* **97:** 298-306.

Pluske, J.R., Williams, I.H. and Aherne, F.X. (1995). Nutrition of the neonatal pig. *In:* The neonatal pig. Development and survival. (Ed. M.A. Varley). CAB International, Wallingford, Oxon, UK, pp. 187-235.

Prosky, L., Asp, N-G., Furda, I., DeVries, J.W., Schweizer, T.F. and Harland, B.F. (1985). Determination of total dietary fiber in foods and food products: Collaborative study. *Journal of the Association of Official Analytical Chemists* **68:** 677-679.

Scheppach, W. (1994). Effects of short chain fatty acids on gut morphology and function. *Gut* **35:** S35-S38.

Schley, P.D. and Field, C.J. (2002). The immune-enhancing effects of dietary fibres and prebiotics. *British Journal of Nutrition* **87** (Suppl 2): S221-230.

Selvendran, R.R. (1984). The plant cell wall as a source of dietary fibre: chemistry and structure. *American Journal of Clinical Nutrition* **39:** 320-337.

Serena, A. and Bach Knudsen, K.E. (2007). Chemical and physicochemical characterisation of co-products from the vegetable food and agro industries. *Animal Feed Science and Technology* **139**:109-124.

Smith, H.W. and Halls, S. (1968). The production of oedema disease and diarrhoea in weaned pigs by the oral administration of *Escherichia coli*: factors that influence the course of the experimental disease. *Journal Medical Microbiology* **1:** 45-59.

Spreeuwenberg, M.A.M., Verdonk, J.M.A.J., Gaskins, H.R. and Verstegen, M.W.A. (2001). Small intestine epithelial barrier function is compromised in pigs with low feed intake at weaning. *Journal of Nutrition* **131:** 1520-1527.

Theander, O., Westerlund, E., Åman, P. and Graham, H. (1989). Plant cell walls and monogastric diets. *Animal Feed Science and Technology* **23:** 205-225.

Theander, O., Åman, P., Westerlund, E. and Graham, H. (1994). Enzymatic/chemical analysis of dietary fiber. *Journal of AOAC International* **77:** 703-709.

Thibault, J-F., Lahaye, M. and Guillon, F. (1992). Physico-chemical properties of food plant cell walls. *In:* Dietary fibre: A component of food: Nutritional function in health and disease. (Eds. T.F. Schweizer and C.A. Edwards). Springer-Verlag, London. pp. 21-39.

Thomsen, L.E., Bach-Knudsen, K.E., Jensen, T.K., Christensen, A.S., Moller, K. and Roepstorff, A. (2007). The effect of fermentable carbohydrates on experimental swine dysentery and whip worm infections in pigs. *Veterinary Microbiology* 119: 152-163.

Van Beers-Schreurs, H.M.G., Nabuurs, M.J.A., Vellenga, L., Kalsbeek-van der Valk, H.J., Wensing, T. and Breukink, H.J. (1998). Weaning and the weanling diet influence the villous height and crypt depth in the small intestine of pigs and alter the concentrations of short-chain fatty acids in the large intestine and blood. *Journal of Nutrition* 128: 947-953.

Van Soest, P.J. (1963). Use of detergents in the analysis of fibrous feeds. II. A rapid method for the determination of fiber and lignin. *Journal of the Association of Official Analytical Chemists* 46: 829-835.

Van Soest, P.J. (1984). Some physical characteristics of dietary fibres and their influence on the microbial ecology of the human colon. *Proceedings of the Nutrition Society* 43: 25-33.

Van Soest, P.J. and Wine, R.H. (1967). Use of detergents in the analysis of fibrous feeds. IV. Determination of plant cell-wall constituents. *Journal of the Association of Official Analytical Chemists* 50: 50-55.

Wellock, I.J., Houdijk, J.G.M. and Kyriazakis, I. (2007) Effect of dietary non-starch polysaccharide solubility and inclusion level on gut health and the risk of post weaning enteric disorders in newly weaned piglets. *Livestock Science* 108: 186-189.

Williams, B.A., Verstegen, M.W.A. and Tamminga, S. (2001). Fermentation in the large intestine of single-stomached animals and its relationship to animal health. *Nutrition Research Reviews* 14: 207-227.

Zoetendal, E.G., Collier, C.T., Koike, S., Mackie, R.I. and Gaskins, H.R. (2004). Molecular ecological analysis of the gastrointestinal microbiota: a review. *Journal of Nutrition* 134: 465-472.

Intestinal balance and equilibrium: setting the scene for health and management

Edwin T. Moran, Jr.
Poultry Science Department, Auburn University, AL 36849, USA

1. Introduction

Nature of the intestine's contents continually changes and a rapid response to optimise its function is paramount. Nutrients vary in type and amount commensurate with diversity of intake, thus, adaptations that accommodate their recovery will favour feed efficiency. In the same respect, threats that impair nutrient access and mucosal integrity must also be rapidly confronted and repaired. Mechanisms are in place to readily adjust pH and provide appropriate amounts of pancreatic enzymes that originate from the wall once gastric digesta enters the small intestine. While such luminal responses are necessary to favourably 'set the scene' for intestinal balance, the greatest part of adjustments for health and management relate to villi lining the surface and their perpetual experience with lumen contents. Villi rapidly alter their number, modulate cell types, and present enzymes commensurate with nutrients at hand while concurrently providing on-going protection. Although rapid accommodation is particularly favourable to animal well-being, its implementation represents an extremely expensive cost to maintain the system. All indications suggest that avian and mammalian species are remarkably similar. The following is an overview of the events and strategy by which the intestine maintains a continual equilibrium with its objective of nutrient recovery. Its breadth necessitates that the author employ 'poetic license' to make regular generalisations in order to communicate the 'big picture'. A wide range of references are provided to support this end.

2. Strategy of nutrient recovery

Comprehending nutrient recovery from the intestinal lumen must precede any understanding of adjustment strategy (Figure 1). Digestion and nutrient absorption by the villus is actually confined its top half where maximal exposure to the lumen exists. This exposure is convectively facilitated by rotation of the shaft using muscle fibers projecting from the *muscularis mucosae* which is

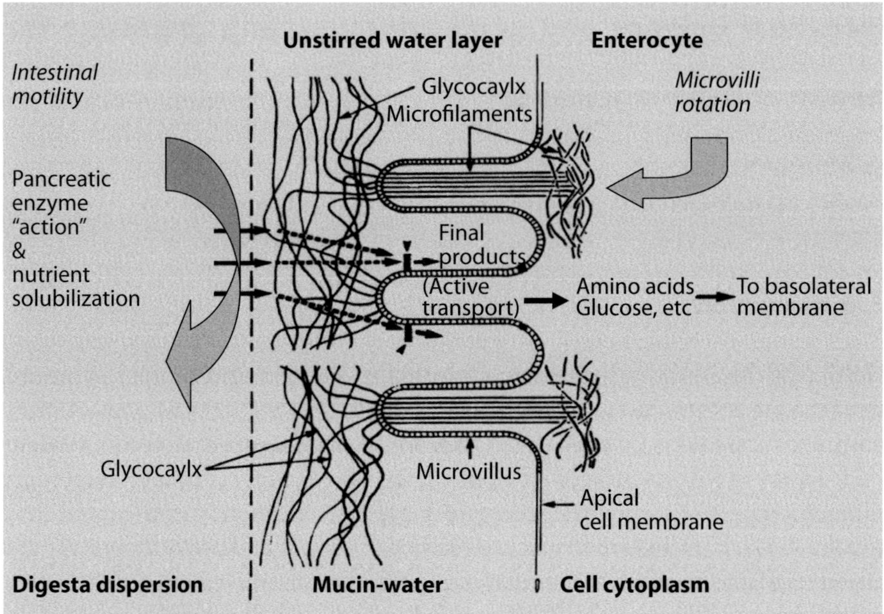

Figure 1. Nutrient recovery is sequentially represented as food macromolecule disassembly in the small intestinal lumen that permits transfer of small secondary products through the unstirred water layer for finalisation of digestion before absorption at the enterocyte surface.

complemented by a concurrent peristalsis originating with the outer circular muscle. Such peristalsis is gently progressive with mammals compared to an enthusiastic reflexive action for fowl. Villi shape may vary from cylindrical to plate or leaf-shaped that in turn influence the dynamics of exposure with motility (Yamauchi and Isshiki, 1991). A mosaic of enterocytes and goblet cells dominates the surface. Microvilli greatly enhance the enterocyte's surface. Each microvillus participates in digestion by employing internal contractile elements to convectively engage enzymes immobilised on the outer membrane with substrates arriving from the lumen (Mooseker and Tilney, 1975; Maroux *et al.*, 1979; Kushak *et al.*, 1981). Differences in enterocyte structure among species are more related to nature of activity than inherent (Michael and Hodges, 1973a). Membrane associated mucin known as the glycocalyx projecting from the microvilli tips has a protein core with large amounts of threonine and serine that are extensively O-glycosylated to give its fibrous character (Gendler and Spicer, 1995; Maury *et al.*, 1995).

Goblet cells are defined by their shape and solely intended to form, store and release secretory mucin (Basbaum, 1985; Koga and Ushiki, 2006; Perez-Vilar, 2007). This mucin also contains a large amounts threonine and serine; however, the polymers are not as extensively O-glycosylated but interlinked and water compatible such that three-dimensional 'fishnet-like' gels form when released (Flood, 1981; Bloomfield, 1983; Sellers *et al.*, 1988; Bansil *et al.*, 1995). 'Entanglement' of the secretory gel with the enterocyte's glycocalyx creates an 'unstirred water layer'. Enzymes immobilised on the microvillus surface are now protected from pancreatic enzymes actively functioning in the lumen while enabling accessibility to their products of reduced size (Nimmerfall and Rosenthaler, 1980; Smithson *et al.*, 1981). Adhering secretory mucin has an extended turn-over time compared to that entering the lumen while pH modifying groups create a favourable surface microclimate (Daniel *et al.*, 1985; Shiau *et al.*, 1985; Pastor *et al.*, 1988; Lehr *et al.*, 1991; Atuma *et al.*, 2001). Microbes in the lumen also have access to pancreatic digesta to compete for nutrient before transfer into the unstirred water layer. Feedstuffs that increase lumen viscosity and impair convection not only provide microbes with a nutritional advantage, but reduced oxygen transfer from the wall alters its partial pressure and nature of membership (Moran, 2006). Microflora are continuously changing in character and threat to the intestine as a result of each animal's total environment and composition of feed (Devrise, 1986; Apajalahti *et al.*, 2004). The intestine's ability to rapidly replace and optimise its surface is expensive, therefore any strategy employed for adaptation must be cost effective (Muramatsu *et al.*, 1987).

3. Crypt multiplication

The initial step in making adjustments to the effective surface involves 'new' cells that collectively originate from a common parent. Stem cell multiplication in the base of each crypt not only gives rise to all cells but may undergo fission and form other crypts and initiate new villi should the need be perceived (Cheng, 1974; Cheng and Leblond, 1974a,b; Loeffler and Grossmann, 1991). Although the small intestine has a common arterial supply, subsequent arteriole subdivisions lead to a partitioning between locations at the mucosa (Figure 2). Crypt cells are separately supplied with fresh blood apart from the villus although they subsequently form a confluence at the villus base before removal in the portal system (Aharinejad *et al.*, 1991). Thus, crypt multiplication depends on arterioles that provide 'basal' levels of nutrients along with oxygen while arterioles supporting digestion-absorption enter at the villus top and

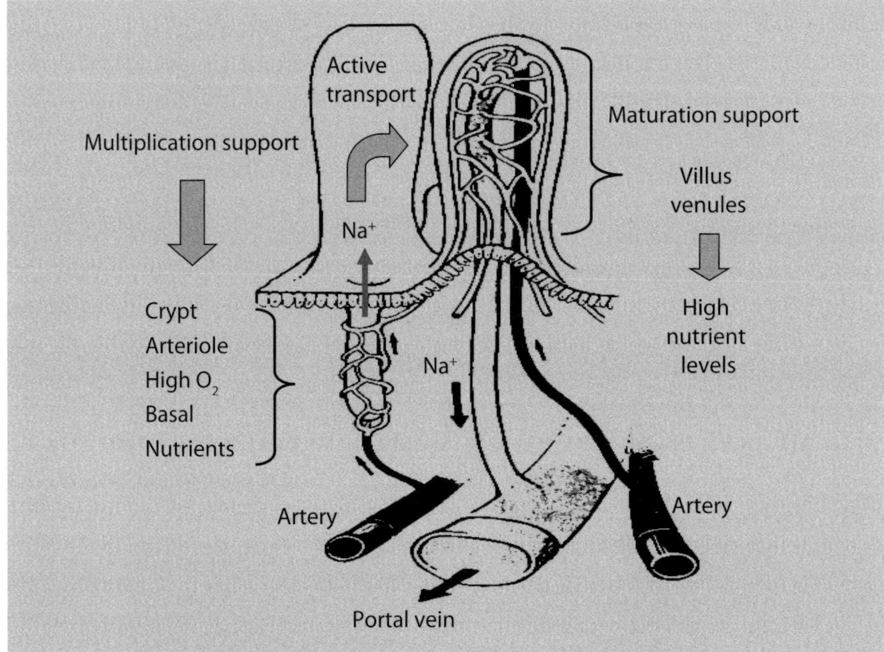

Figure 2. Arterioles in the small intestinal mucosa subdivide and separately supply the crypt versus villus. Villus entry occurs at the top to remove absorbed nutrients before progressing down the shaft and convergence with flow from the crypt and portal return. Imperfections in the crypt enable sodium to enter the lumen and support active transport. Passage of absorbed nutrients adjacent to maturing enterocytes supports a continuation of their development. (Adapted and redrawn from Aharinejad et al.*, 1991).*

convey nutrients to the base (Alpers, 1972; Kaut and Potten, 1986). Either energy, protein or their combination if either lacking or superfluous can affect the dynamics of cell multiplication in the crypt and subsequently alter villus length as well as number (figure 3). Nutritional support appears to alter the rate of renewal largely by modulating duration of the synthetic phase in the cell multiplication cycle (Rose *et al.*, 1971; Koga and Kimura, 1979, 1980). Frequent cell multiplication also necessitates a minimisation of 'tight junctions', therefore crypt integrity is lacking. Associated 'leakage' into the lumen appears to provide sodium as a requisite for active transport before re-entry into the portal system and cycle completion (Madara and Trier, 1982).

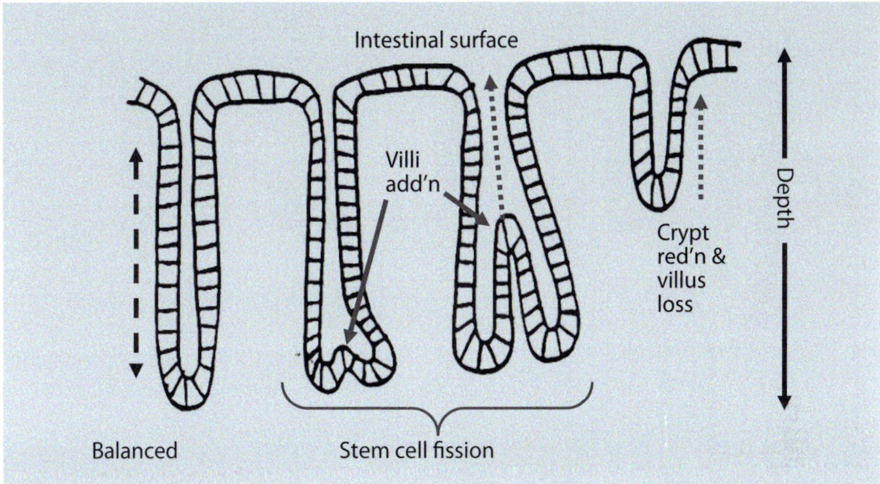

Figure 3. Stem cell dynamics in the crypt determines the extent of cell replacement and whether villi are formed or lost. Overall activity is related to nutritional support as conveyed by vascular information corresponding to the body at-large rather than nutrient levels from the villus that parallels food in the lumen.

4. Establishing enterocyte-goblet cells

Once cells generated in the crypt exit at the base of the villus, enterocyte and goblet cell characteristics become more histologically discernable (Figure 4). Reproductive capacity of these pre-enterocytes and pre-goblet cells continues for several cycles before ceasing and commitment to one cell type of the other is established. During this transient period of multiplication and 'decision', cells structurally indicative as pre-enterocytes may be 'converted' to pre-goblet cells allowing adjustments to the final relationship of one to the other to change as 'conditions' dictate (Kurosumi *et al.*, 1981). Perhaps the fixing of an enterocyte: goblet cell ratio at the same location as the confluence of flow from crypt and upper villus is not coincidental. Associated vascular conditions could best convey existing terms and expected needs over the next one to two days.

5. Surface maturation

Once committed, pre-enterocytes and pre-goblet cells located at the base of the villus must progress to the top and assume features necessary to participate in nutrient recovery. Formation of microvilli, insertion of surface enzymes,

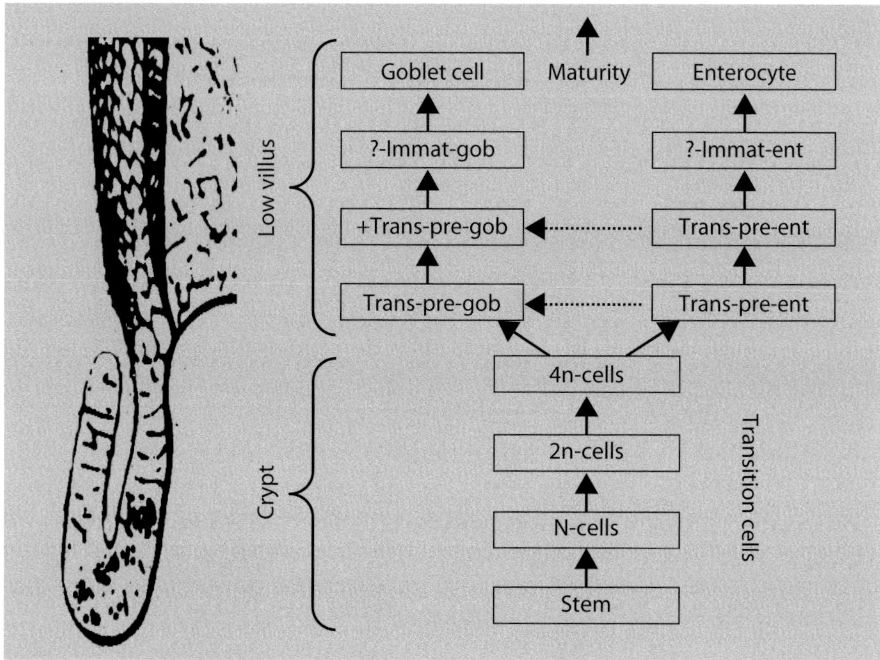

Figure 4. Transition cells arising from multiplication in the crypt exit at the villus base where a convergence of vessels from crypt-villus-GALT appears to influence their functional commitment to either being an enterocyte or goblet cell. Multiple sources of information at this location also enable each cell to modify its activity, surface characteristics, and enzyme profile to accommodate nutrient recovery and protection in the foreseeable future.

and addition of a glycocalyx network corresponding to a functional surface dominates change with enterocyte maturity (Altmond and Leblond, 1982; Naim *et al.*, 1999; Fan *et al.*, 2001). Goblet cell transition involves an enhanced mucin production which is changing from a neutral to acidic character (Umesaki *et al.*, 1982; More *et al.*, 1987; Chambraud *et al.*, 1989; Paulus *et al.*, 1993). Structure of the vascular system is not only expected to be central to nutrient recovery but subsequently support new cells in their various stages of maturation. Essentially, arterial blood first provides villus top with oxygen to support active transport then accepts absorbed nutrients before passing adjacent to developing enterocytes en route to the base (Komuro and Hashimoto, 1990; Aharinejad *et al.*, 1991). Nutrient exposure at this time likely influences extent of enzyme expression in anticipation of future needs (Wilson, 1984; Beaulieu *et al.*, 1989; Huerou-Luron, 2002). Intensity of digestive-absorptive activity further determines cell life span and total surface competent to do so (Michael and Hodges, 1973b; Komai and Kimura, 1979; Kojima *et al.*, 1993).

6. Protection

Gut associated lymphoid tissue located at the mucosal surface and in the lamina propria provide a continuum of secretory IgA for surface protection as the animal's experiences accrue (Rojas and Apodaca, 2002; Vaughn *et al.*, 2006). Intimate contact of vascular flow from mucosal lymphoid tissue to the confluence of villus-crypt provides a particularly convenient access to convey immediate experiences. Immunoglobulin uptake near the crypts with their eventual externalisation upon maturation provides a fixed area at the surface with protection. Extrusion of senescent cells from the villi tip and their subsequent disintegration permits scavenging of the lumen of the 'freed' IgA (Holman, 1975; Potten and Allen, 1977). Any immunoglobulin mosaic based on a composite of mucosal experience reduces threats accordingly, but costs associated with its maintenance escalate as well (King *et al.*, 2005).

7. Summary

Adaptation of the small intestine to the continuum of changes that occur in the lumen primarily involves the villus. This accommodation encompasses alteration of their number in the wall, modulation of surface exposure, synchronisation of digestive enzymes with food at hand, and surface protection. Crypt stem cells not only act as source for the entire covering of the villus, but provide for either expanding or contracting their density in the wall. Arterioles supplying the crypt and villus differ to support divergent activities. Crypt vessels convey nutrients and information to alter cell multiplication commensurate with the animal's well-being as a whole. Villus arteriole entry at its apex and flow down the outer surface removes nutrients and these subsequently support immature cells through progressive states of development. Cells exiting the crypt at the base of the villus encounter blood converging from the crypt and upper villus. This diverse information is used to establish a most favourable enterocyte-goblet cell relationship, provide the best array of digestive enzyme to meet anticipated needs while receiving immunoglobulins for insertion and protection. A 'rolling' three day turnover permits continual and rapid adaptation at any one location along the intestine. Maintaining an intestinal system acute to change is essential for optimal animal performance and health.

References

Aharinejad, S., Lametschwandtner, A., Franz, P. and Firbas, W. (1991) The vascularization of the digestive tract studied by scanning electron microscopy with special emphasis on the teeth, esophagus, stomach, small and large intestine, pancreas, and liver. *Scanning Microscopy* **5**: 811-849.

Alpers, D.H. (1972). Protein synthesis in intestinal mucosa: the effect of route of Administration of precursor amino acids. *The Journal of Clinical Investigation* **51:** 167-173.

Apajalahti, J., Kettunen, A. and Graham, H. (2004). Characteristics of the gastrointestinal Microbial communities, with special reference to the chicken. *World's Poultry Science Association* **60:** 223-232.

Altmann, G.G., and Leblond, C.P. (1982). Changes in the size and structure of the Nucleolus of columnar cells during their migration from crypt base to villus top in rat jejunum. *Journal of Cell Science* **56**: 83-99.

Atuma, C., Strugala, V., Allen, A., and Holm, L. (2001). The adherent gastrointestinal mucus gel layer: thickness and physical state in vivo. *American Journal of Physiology Gastrointestinal and Liver Physiology* **280**: G922-G-929.

Altmond, G.G. and Leblond, C.P. (1982). Changes in the size and structure of the Nucleolus of columnar cells during their migration from crypt base to villus top in rat jejunum. *Journal of Cell Science* **56:** 83-99.

Bansil, R., Stanley, E. and LaMont, J.T. (1995). Mucin biophysics. *Annual Review of Physiology* **57:** 635-657.

Basbaum, C. (1985). Regulation of mucus secretion in the intestine. *Gastroenterology Clinical Biology* **9:** 45-47.

Beaulieu, J.-F., Nichols, B. and Quaroni, A. (1989). Post-translational regulation of sucrase-isomaltase expression in intestinal crypt and villus cells. *Journal of Biological Chemistry* **264:** 20000-20011.

Bloomfield, V.A. (1983). Hydrodynamic properties of mucus glycoproteins. *Biopolymers* **22:** 2141-2141.

Chambraud, L., Bernadac, A., Gorvel, J.-P. and Maroux, S. (1989). Renewal of goblet cell mucus granules during cell migration along the crypt-villus axis in rabbit jejunum: an immunolabeling study. *Biology of the Cell* **65:** 151-162.

Cheng, H. (1974). Origin, differentiation and renewal of the four main epithelial cell types of the mouse small intestine II. Mucous cells. *American Journal of Anatomy* **141:** 481-502.

Cheng, H. and Leblond, C.P. (1974a). Origin, differentiation and renewal of the four main epithelial cell types in the mouse small intestine I. Columnar cell. *American Journal of Anatomy* **141:** 461-480.

Cheng, H. and Leblond, C.P. (1974b). Origin, differentiation and renewal of the four main epithelial cell types in the mouse small intestine V. Uniterian theory of the origin of the four epithelial cell types. *American Journal of Anatomy* **141:** 537-562.

Daniel, H., Neugebauer, B., Kratz, A. and Rehner, G. (1985). Localization of acid microclimate along intestinal villi of rat jejunum. *American Journal of Anatomy.* **248** (*Gastrointestinal and Liver Physiology* **11**)**:** G293-G298.

Devrise, L. (1986). Importance of the intestinal bacterial flora of poultry II. Effects on intestinal function and artificial modification of the gut flora. *Vlaams Diergeneeskundig Tijdschrift* **55:** 357-368.

Fan, M.Z., Stoll, B., Jiang, R. and Burrin, D.G. (2001). Enterocyte digestive activity along the crypt-villus and longitudinal axes in the neonatal pig small intestine. *Journal of Animal Science* **79:** 371-381.

Flood, P.R. (1981). On the ultrastructure of mucus. *Biomedical Research* **2** (Suppl): 49-52.

Gendler, J.G. and Spicer, A.P. (1995). Epithelial mucin genes. *Annual Review of Physiology* **57:** 607-634.

Holman, J. (1975). Fine structural changes of senescent enterocytes in the extrusion zone of chicken intestinal villi. *Acta Veterinaria Brno* **44:** 3-8.

Huerou-Luron, I.L. (2002). Production and gene expression of brush border disaccharides and peptidases during development in pigs and calves. In: *Biology of the Intestine in Growing Animals* (Eds. R. Zabielski, P.C. Gregory and B. Westrom. Elsevier Science. B.V. pp. 491-513.

Kaut, P. and Potten, C.S. (1986). Effects of puromycin, cycloheximide and noradrenaline on cell migration within the crypts and on villi of the small intestine. *Cell & Tissue Kinetics* **19:** 611-625.

King, M.R., Ravindran, V., Morel, P.C.H., Thomas, D.V., Birtles, M.J. and Pluske, J.R. (2005). Effects of spray-dried colostrum and plasma on the performance and gut morphology of broiler chickens. *Australian Journal of Agricultural Research* **56:** 811-817.

Koga, A. and Kimura, S. (1979). Influence of restricted diet on the cell renewal of the mouse small intestine. *Journal of Nutritional Science and Vitaminology* **25**: 265-267.

Koga, A. and Kimura, S. (1980). Influence of restricted diet on the cell cycle in the crypt of the mouse small intestine. *Journal of Nutritional Science and Vitaminology* **26:** 33-38.

Koga, D., and Ushiki, T. (2006). Three-dimensional ultrastructure of the golgi apparatus In different cells: high-resolution scanning electron microscopy of osmium-macerated tissues. *Archives of Histology and Cytology* **69**: 357-374.

Kojima, A., Kasai, S., and Suga-Katayama, Y. (1993). Recovery of the ultrastructure of jejunal absorptive cells and absorption of nutrients in starved then re-fed rat. *Journal of Nutritional Science and Vitaminology* **39**: 23-32.

Komai, M. and Kimura, S. (1979). Effects of restricted diet and intestinal flora on the life span of small intestine epithelial cells in mice. *Journal of Nutritional Science and Vitaminology* **25:** 87-94.

Komuro, T. and Hashimoto, Y. (1990). Three-dimensional structure of the rat intestinal wall (mucosa and submucosa). *Archives of Histology and Cytology* **53:** 1-21.

Kurosumi, K., Shibuichi, I. and Tosaka, H. (1981). Transition between columnar absorptive cells and goblet cells in the rat jejunal epithelium. *Archivium histologicum japonicum* **44:** 405-427.

Kushak, R., Ozols, A., Antonyuk, Z., Gailite, B., Tarvid, I., Sheshukova, T., and Nasurlaeva, I. (1981). Relationship of intrinsic enzymes of the apical glycocalyx and mucosa of the small intestine of chicks. *Comparative Biochemistry and Physiology* **70**: 107-109.

Lehr, C.-M., Poelma, F.G.J., Junginger, H.E., and Tukker, J.J. (1991). An estimate of turnover time of intestinal mucus gel layer in the rat in situ loop. *International Journal of Phamaceutics* **70**: 235-240.

Loeffler, M. and Grossman, B. (1991). A stochastic model with formation of subunits applied to the growth of intestinal crypts. *Journal of Theoretical Biology* **150:** 175-191.

Madara, J.L. and Trier, J.S. (1982). Structure and permeability of goblet cell tight junctions in rat small intestine. *Journal of Membrane Biology* **66:** 145-157.

Maroux, S., Louvard, D., Semeriva, M., and Desnuelle, P. (1979). Hydrolase bound to the intestinal brush border: An example of transmembrane proteins. *Ann. Biol. Anim. Bioch. Biophys.* **19**: 787-790.

Maury, J., Nicoletti, C. and Guzzo-Chambraud, L. (1995). The filamentous brush border Glycocalyx, a mucin-like marker of enterocyter hyper-polarization. *European Journal of Biochemistry* **228:** 323-331.

Michael, E. and Hodges, R.D. (1973a). Structure and histochemistry of the normal intestine of the fowl. I. The mature absorptive cell. *Histochemical Journal* **5:** 313-333.

Michael, E. and Hodges, R.D. (1973b). Histochemical changes in the fowl small intestine associated with enhanced absorption after feed restriction. *Society of Histochemistry* **36:** 39-49.

Mooseker, M.S. and Tilney, L.G. (1975). Organization of an actin filament-membrane complex. Filament polarity and membrane attachment in the microvilli of intestinal epithelial cells. *Journal of Cell Biology* **67:** 725-743.

Moran, E.T., Jr. (2006). Anatomy, microbes, and fiber: Small versus large intestine. *Journal of Applied Poultry Research* **15:** 154-160.

More, J., Fioramonti, J., Benazet, F. and Bueno, L. (1987) Histochemical characterization of glycoproteins present in jejunal and colonic goblet cells of pigs on different diets. A biopsy study using chemical methods and peroxidase-labelled lectins. *Histochemistry* **87:** 189-194.

Muramatsu, T., Takasu, O., Furuse, M., Tasaki, I. and Okimura, J.-I. (1987). Influence of the gut microflora on protein synthesis in tissues and in the whole body of chicks. *Biochemical Journal* **246:** 475-479.

Naim, H.Y., Joberty, G., Alfalah, M. and Jacob, R. (1999) Temporal association of the N- and O-linked glycosylation events and their implication in the polarized sorting of intestinal brush border sucrase-isomaltase, aminopeptidase N, and dipeptidyl peptidase IV. *Journal of Biological Chemistry* **274:** 17961-17967.

Nimmerfall, F. and Rosenthaler, J. (1980). Significance of goblet-cell mucin layer, the outermost luminal barrier to passage through the gut wall. *Biochemical and Biophysical Research Communications* **94:** 960-966.

Pastor, L.M., Ballesta, J., Madrid, J.F., Perz-Tomas, R., and Hernandez, F. (1988). A histochemical study of the mucins in the digestive tract of the chicken. *Acta Histochemica* **83**: 91-97.

Paulus, U., Loeffler, M., Zeidler, J., Owen, G. and Potten, C.S. (1993). The differentiation and lineage development of goblet cells in the murine small intestinal crypt: experimental and modeling studies. *Journal of Cell Science* **106:** 473-484.

Perez-Vilar, J. (2007). Mucin granule intraluminal organization. *American Journal of Respiratory Cell and Molecular Biology* **36**: 183-190.

Potten, C.S. and Allen, T.D. (1977). Ultrastructure of cell loss in intestinal mucosa. *Journal of Ultrastructural Resolution* **60:** 272-277.

Rojas, R., and Apodaca, G. (2002). Immunoglobin transport across polarized epithelial cells. *Molecular Biology* **3:** 944-955.

Rose, P.M., Hopper, A.F. and Wannemacher, Jr, R.W. (1971). Cell population changes in the intestinal mucosa of protein-depleted or starved rats I. Changes in mitotic cycle time. *Journal of Cell Biology* **50:** 887-892.

Sellers, L.A., Allen, A., Morris, E.R. and Ross-Murphy, S.B. (1988). Mucus glycoprotein gels. Role of glycoprotein polymeric structure and carbohydrate side-chains in gel-formation. *Carbohydrate Research* **178:** 93-110.

Shiau, Y.-F., Fernandez, P., Jackson, M.J., and McMonagle, S. (1985). Mechanisms maintaining a low-pH microclimate in the intestine. *American Journal of Anatomy.* **248** (*Gastrointestinal and Liver Physiology* **11**): G608-G617.

Smithson, K.W., Jacobs, L.R., and Gray, G.M. (1981). Intestinal diffusion barrier: unstirred water layer or membrane surface mucous coat? *Science* **214**: 1241-1243.

Umesaki, Y., Sakata, T. and Yajima, T. (1982). Abrupt induction of GDP-fucose: asiol GM1 fucosyltransferase in the small intestine after conventionalization of germ-free mice. *Biochemical and Biophysical Research Communications* **105:** 439-443.

Vaughn, L.E., Holt, P.S., Moore, R.W. and Mast, R.K. (2006). Enhanced gross visualization of chicken peyer's patch: novel staining technique applied to fresh tissue specimens. *Avian Diseases* **50:** 298-302.

Wilson, J.R., Dworaczyk, D.A. and Weiser, M.W. (1984). Intestinal epithelial cell differentiation-related changes in glycosyltransferase activities in rats. *Biochimica et Biophysica Acta* **797:** 396-376.

Yamauchi, K.-E. and Isshiki, Y. (1991). Scanning electron microscopic observations on the intestinal villi in growing white leghorn and broiler chickens from 1 to 30 days of age. *British Poultry Science* **32:** 67-78.

Managing disease resistance: applying advanced methods to understand gastrointestinal microbial communities

Margie D. Lee
Dept. Population Health, Poultry Diagnostic and Research Center, The University of Georgia, Athens GA 30602, USA

1. Introduction to the intestinal microbiota

A resurgence of interest in the behaviour of commensal bacteria in the intestine has lead to a remarkable transformation in our view of how bacteria participate in intestinal health. Studies investigating these effects have resulted in microbiologists, developmental biologists, animal scientists and veterinarians integrating biochemistry, cell biology, molecular biology, and ecology in an approach to determine how animals develop and mature. The findings are welcomed as timely additions to our present quest to optimise antibiotic-free animal production. They are also crucial for designing and understanding the mechanisms of action of prebiotics, probiotics and direct-fed microbials in animal health. The intestinal microbiota is part of a complex ecosystem that affects animal health and performance through its effects on gut morphology, nutrition, and the immune response. The most commonly used modulators of gastrointestinal microbial ecology are prebiotics, probiotics and growth-promoting antibiotics. However, the use of antibiotics in meat and poultry production has become very controversial and many poultry integrators have reduced their use. Integrators have experienced limited success in producing antibiotic-free birds because of the resulting increase in clostridial enteropathies. Prebiotics, probiotics and direct-fed microbials have been used to facilitate formation of a mature intestine and to prevent development of enteritis. In order to successfully utilise these products, and develop more effective formulations, we must first understand how the intestinal microbiota contributes to intestinal health.

1.1. Commercial background

In 1997, countries within the European Union began banning the use of subtherapeutic antibiotics (also known as antibiotic-growth promotants) in meat and poultry production; 2006 marks the new era of 'antibiotic-free' production in the EU. Consequently the prevalence of necrotic enteritis and dysbacteriosis has also increased in poultry. Necrotic enteritis, first described in 1961, is caused by toxigenic strains of *Clostridium perfringens* (Parish, 1961). Until recently the disease was infrequently diagnosed in commercial production, presumably because of the disease preventing qualities of continuously-fed low dose antibiotics. Dysbacteriosis is a new enteric syndrome, described in the EU following the growth-promotant ban. Another form of subclinical necrotic enteritis is hepatitis and cholangiohepatitis found in broilers at processing. It has been estimated that broiler flocks in Norway had losses due to hepatitis condemnations as great as 20% (Schaller *et al.*, 1998). The subclinical forms of clostridial enteropathies may be most economically important because they impair the feed conversion ratio in broilers (Williams *et al.*, 2005, Van Immerseel *et al.*, 2004). Therefore the increasing prevalence of subclinical necrotic enteritis and dysbacteriosis are the most significant challenge to organic and antibiotic-free poultry production in the world (Lu *et al.*, 2006; Williams *et al.*, 2005; Van Immerseel *et al.*, 2004).

2. Necrotic enteritis

Issues relevant to the prevalence of necrotic enteritis and related syndromes have been recently reviewed (Williams *et al.*, 2005; Van Immerseel *et al.*, 2004). *C. perfringens* is a nearly ubiquitous spore-forming anaerobic bacterium that can be readily found in soil, dust, faeces, feed, poultry litter and intestinal contents. Therefore, young chicks are exposed to the pathogen at a very early age. However, clinical disease does not occur until the birds are 3-4 weeks of age. Several studies have demonstrated that diet composition is a contributing factor; high levels of animal by-products such as fishmeal, wheat, barley, oats, or rye, have been shown to correlate with a higher prevalence of disease. Therefore those regions that feed wheat or large amounts of fishmeal have more frequent and severe disease than areas feeding a corn/maize based ration. Also, conditions that result in damage to the intestinal mucosa or disturbance to the normal intestinal microbiota appear to predispose birds to the disease. For example, coccidiosis caused by *Eimeria*-infections of the intestine, predisposes broiler chickens to *C. perfringens*-mediated necrotic enteritis (Wages and Opengart, 2003); thus coccidiosis control is important. Ionophore antibiotics (such as monensin), organic arsenicals, and vaccines are used in poultry production in an attempt to reduce coccidiosis but these treatments do not completely eliminate the parasites. Therefore, clinical symptoms of clostridial enteropathy may result from a proliferation of *Clostridium* in the small intestine in response to mucosal damage by other enteric parasites; however changing environmental conditions may also stimulate toxin secretion by the *C. perfringens* that are already present.

2.1. *Clostridium* toxicity

Clostridia are a diverse group of anaerobic bacteria that primarily acquire energy by hydrolysing macromolecules such proteins, lipids, and carbohydrates. They are found in many environments and are common members of the intestinal microbiota of most animals (Collins *et al.*, 1994). The pathogenic *Clostridium* species are notable because of their ability to produce disease in many different species of animals and because they can produce a variety of toxins. The cytotoxic activities of pathogenic species have been well studied (Rood, 1998; Karasawa *et al.*, 2003). *C. perfringens* is particularly interesting in that the type of disease it causes and the host species affected, is dependant upon its array of toxins (Petit *et al.*, 1999). For example the α-toxin is important for the pathogenesis of gangrene in humans and necrotic enteritis in chickens; however additional toxins are needed to produce necrotic enteritis in lambs, piglets, and calves. The toxins of pathogenic *Clostridium* are often enzymes that exhibit enzymatic activity targeting host macromolecules. For example, the α-toxin of *C. perfringens* is a phospholipase C (also known as lecithinase) that has substrate specificity for sphingomyelin, a phospholipid that is a major component of vertebrate cell membranes (Petit *et al.*, 1999; Rood, 1998). The phospholipase C activity of the α-toxin is also responsible for the haemolytic colonies characteristic of pathogenic isolates of *C. perfringens* (Clark *et al.*, 2003).

Toxin expression assays, genomic studies, and structural analysis of the promoter region of the α-toxin indicate that the gene encoding the toxin is regulated (Petit *et al.*, 1999; Rood, 1998). At least two loci, including a putative two-component regulatory system, have been shown to affect toxin expression however environmental signals that affect toxin production have not been identified (Rood, 1998). Toxin expression is affected by growth phase; production is optimal during exponential growth and decreases with the onset of the stationary phase. Bacteria possess intricate systems for detecting nutrient levels in the environment and adjust their metabolism to adapt to changes in food sources, temperature and environmental stressors. They produce signalling molecules as part of a quorum-sensing system that allows monitoring of cell density in the community. Growth-phase regulation of α–toxin expression suggests that intercellular signalling may be involved and indeed quorum-sensing has been shown to influence α-toxin production in *C. perfringens* (Ohtani *et al.*, 2002). Quorum sensing enables individual bacterial cells to communicate with many different members of the microbiota because many bacterial species excrete common quorum-sensing molecules. For example, quorum-sensing LuxS homologues have been found in gram-positive (including *C. perfringens*) and gram-negative bacteria that reside in diverse environments. Therefore, in addition to detecting nutrient levels and environmental stressors, bacteria can also detect whether the overall bacterial community has gained or lost density and may be able to respond to changes in community composition. While lesions associated with necrotic enteritis has been attributed to toxin production from an overgrowth of *C. perfringens*, the composition and density of the intestinal community may also be a trigger that induces the production of toxin.

3. Commensal bacteria

There are over a trillion bacteria within the intestine of a vertebrate animal; 10 times the number of host cells (Drasar and Barrow, 1985). The composition of this normal intestinal microbial community plays an important role in animal health and performance through its effect on gut morphology, nutrition, pathogenesis of intestinal disease and the immune response (Falk *et al.*, 2000). Many of the early studies that evaluated the effects of intestinal bacteria were done using gnotobiotic (germ-free) animals (Gordon and Pesti, 1972). These studies were particularly illuminating because the development of gastrointestinal function, devoid of commensal and pathogenic bacteria, could be described. For example, germ-free animals require more calories in order to have comparable weight gains as conventional animals. In addition, the intestines of germ-free animals were found to be relatively underdeveloped and poorly innervated (Xu and Gordon, 2003). Therefore, performance and morphometric comparisons, such as villus height and size of cecum, clearly showed that commensal bacteria could be beneficial. Moreover, rats fed a vitamin-deficient diet could rely completely on their intestinal microbiota for production of vitamins K, B, and E while germ-free rats displayed clinical symptoms of vitamin deficiency unless they were reconstituted with normal microbiota (Draser and Barrow, 1985). These studies inspired a quest to characterise and identify the beneficial bacteria; for example the Schaedler intestinal consortium has been used in many studies to describe the benefits of commensal intestinal bacteria (Schaedler *et al.*, 1965).

3.1. Intestinal development

The bacterial community is now regarded as a multicellular, multifunctional organ whose genomes provide metabolic functions that the host has not yet acquired or evolved in its own genome (Xu and Gordon, 2003). In addition to providing the ability to hydrolyse complex plant polysaccharides, particularly important in ruminant nutrition, some members provide the important function of vitamin biosynthesis. Studies investigating how bacteria contribute to the development of host intestinal function are now underway and have revealed a surprisingly symbiotic relationship. Reconstituting the intestinal microbiota of gnotobiotic mice has shown that bacteria can also direct postnatal development of the intestine. Xu and Gordon (2003) recently reviewed the literature regarding the intestinal microbial community as part of a series of Inaugural Articles by members of the National Academy of Sciences. This review, entitled 'Honor thy Symbionts' illustrated the changing attitudes regarding intestinal bacteria. For example, *Bacteroides thetaiotaomicron* has multiple effects on intestinal development. When used to reconstitute gnotobiotic mice, it is able to enhance development of the intestinal submucosal capillary beds. The capillary network is rudimentary in adult gnotobiotic mice, however when the mice are colonised with *B. thetaiotaomicron,* angiogenesis is stimulated (Stappenbeck *et al.*, 2002). This finding indicates that certain commensal bacteria may be necessary for development of the intestine to its full absorptive capacity. *B. thetaiotaomicron* also directs increased expression of terminal α-linked fucose by enterocytes positioned in the distal small intestine (Bry *et al.*, 1996). These changes in host glycan expression allow the bacterium to expand its colonisation niche to additional areas along the small intestine. Colonisation of the small intestine with this potential 'symbiont' also augments colonisation by other commensal members of the microbiota. These results suggest that the development of colonisation niches and the behaviour of pathogens may be influenced by the early development of the intestinal microbiota.

3.2. Probiotics and pathogen resistance

One of the most important functions of the intestinal microbiota is to suppress pathogenic populations of bacteria. Until recently, suppression was assumed to occur because the interaction of bacteria in the intestines is fundamentally competitive. Nutrient utilisation, enhanced by complementary interspecies metabolic activity and production of inhibitory metabolites, can produce a community that is resistant to colonisation by pathogens. However resistance to some enteropathogens may be enhanced in animals by early exposure to intestinal 'symbionts' that direct the nutrient foundation of the developing intestine and foster development of intestinal microbiota that suppress the growth or toxin production of enteropathogens. This hypothesis is supported by published studies. Fukata *et al.* (1991) showed that germ-free birds which were reconstituted with either *Lactobacillus* or *Enterococcus* were more resistant to colonisation with *C. perfringens*. This finding indicates competitive suppression, however Craven *et al.* (1999) demonstrated that probiotic administration reduced α-toxin production by *C. perfringens* in the chicken intestine. These findings suggest that the composition of the community influences the pathogenesis of necrotic enteritis. Furthermore, probiotics have been shown to reduce the prevalence and severity of necrotic enteritis lesions in chickens (Hofacre *et al.*, 1998a,b; Kaldhusdal *et al.*, 2001; Decroos *et al.*, 2004).

3.3. Intestinal protection by microbiota

Some members of the intestinal bacterial community also exhibit anti-inflammatory effects on the mucosa (Rafter, 2002; Madden and Hunter, 2002). Neish (2002) described a mechanism by which some bacterial proteins act as inhibitors of the NF-κB inflammation activation pathway. Neish, an epithelial pathologist, sought to explain why some salmonellae failed to cause mucosal inflammation despite the fact that they were able to invade epithelial cells. In these studies, proteins of proinflammatory bacteria (pathogens) stimulated the NF-κB pathway resulting in IL-8 secretion by epithelial cells and mucosal inflammation. Some pathogens can also inhibit the NF-κB pathway by inhibiting IκB ubiquitination (Neish *et al.*, 2000). This area of research has resulted in an emerging class of putative ubiquitin-like proteases that are believed to have a dual function of processing ubiquitin-like molecules for the microbe and altering host cellular proteins. Ubiquitin-like proteases are theorised to be used by commensal intestinal bacteria in order to blockade the NF-κB pathway and reduce host response to their presence (Neish *et al.*, 2000). These studies demonstrate the positive effects of some members of the bacterial intestinal community. An aberrant host response to the intestinal microbiota is thought to contribute to the development of a number of inflammatory intestinal diseases as well as some intestinal cancers (Rafter, 2002; Madden and Hunter, 2002; Neish *et al.*, 2000). Bacterial communities primarily composed of lactobacilli and bifidobacteria may reduce the prevalence and severity of these maladies. However, in order to assess the mechanisms involved in stabilisation of the intestinal microbiota, we must identify the major players in the ecological development of the intestinal bacterial community.

4. Analysis of intestinal bacterial communties

4.1. Analytical methods

Compositional analysis of intestinal bacterial communities is also increasing in interest, partly fuelled by new technologies that enable broad surveys of diverse environments. Currently there are 2 methods used to assay the composition of microbial communities. The culture method is recognised to have significant weaknesses due to the inability to culture many of the abundant organisms in some environmental samples (Amann *et al.*, 1995). Less than 10% of the intestinal bacterial population can be characterised by current cultivation procedures (Draser and Barrow, 1985; Amann *et al.*, 1995). Therefore our limited view of intestinal ecology is biased due to the selective nature of artificial culture. For many habitats, it has been shown that direct microscopic counts, even those including viability stains, exceed culture-based viable-cell counts by many orders of magnitude (Amann *et al.*, 1995). Staley and Konopka coined the phrase 'great plate count anomaly' to describe this phenomenon which has been recognised since the advent of microbiology (Staley and Konopka *et al.*, 1985). Therefore, molecular techniques that do not rely on cultivation procedures have been found to be more reliable in evaluating the microbial ecology of many ecosystems including the intestine. A molecular method, analysis of small subunit (ssu or 16S) rRNA genes present among the community DNA, is currently used because of this gene's discriminatory ability in identifying bacteria to the genus, and frequently species, level (Amann *et al.*, 1995). Fluorescence in situ hybridisation, using group-specific or species-specific 16S rDNA oligonucleotide probes, is useful for visualising the presence, spatial organisation, and composition of a microbial community. However, prior knowledge is needed in order to select discriminatory probes that hybridise to the most abundant bacteria in the community (Amann *et al.*, 1995) therefore the composition can be revealed by sequencing cloned PCR amplicons resulting from targeting the 16S rRNA genes present in the metagenome of the microbial community (Suau *et al.*, 1999). 16S rDNA libraries can be invaluable for sampling the composition of bacterial communities, especially those that are composed of organisms that are difficult to cultivate. Several other techniques have been developed to detect changes in the diversity of bacterial communities; these rely on characterising DNA sequence variability of amplified 16S rRNA as displayed in denaturing gradient gel electrophoresis (Zoetendal *et al.*, 1998; Simpson *et al.*, 1999), temperature gradient gel electrophoresis (Zoetendal *et al.*, 1998), and terminal restriction fragment length polymorphisms (T-RFLP) (Avaniss-Aghajani *et al.*, 1994). These methods are rapid and simple to perform but assigning bacterial identity to the bands and quantitatively interpreting the bacterial community change is quite complex (Kitts, 2001).

4.2. Recent studies

Studies based on the culturable bacteria microbiota of chickens have been extensively conducted over the past 40 years. The predominant culturable bacteria detected in the chicken cecum have been obligate anaerobes at the level of 10^{11} per gram of content (Barnes *et al.*, 1972). At least 38 different types of anaerobic bacteria have been isolated from the chicken cecum (Barnes, 1979) composed of more than 200 different bacterial strains (Mead, 1989). Mead found the gram-positive cocci (*Peptostreptococcus*) composed 28% of the total culturable bacteria, *Bacteroidaceae* (20%), *Eubacterium* spp. (16%), *Bifidobacterium* spp. (9%), budding cocci (6%), *Gemmiger formicilis* (5%), and *Clostridium* spp. (5%) (Mead, 1989). However, the authors estimated that only 10 - 60% of the total bacteria in the cecum were detected by culture (Barnes *et al.*, 1972; Barnes, 1979; Salanitro *et al.*, 1974).

Although there are limitations of molecular methods such as PCR in providing accurate quantitative measurements of the actual composition of a microbial community (Farrelly *et al.*, 1995; Suzuki and Giovannoni, 1996), recent studies of the chicken intestine have produced remarkably similar results to the cultivation studies. Gong *et al.* (2002) used a combination of culture, 16S rDNA libraries and 16S rDNA-T-RFLP (terminal restriction fragment length polymorphism) to characterise the bacterial community of the cecum of 6 week-old broiler chickens that were fed a corn-soy diet without growth promotants. The most abundant group comprising the libraries were the low G+C gram-positives (*Clostridium* and *Ruminococcus*) and *Fecalobacterium (Fusobacterium) prausnitzii*. Similar results were reported by Zhu *et al.* (2002) using 16S rDNA libraries and TTGE (temperature gradient gel electrophoresis) to study the microbiota of broiler chickens fed a corn-soy diet that contained animal protein and an anticoccidial compound. *Clostridia* were the dominant group however they reported that 40% of the library sequences were related to *Sporomusa* or enterics related to the γ-Proteobacteria, such as *E. coli*.

Several studies have also addressed the composition of the chicken small intestinal microbiota and have revealed a surprisingly diverse bacterial community (Knarreborg *et al.*, 2002; Van der Wielen *et al.*, 2002; Lu *et al.*, 2003). These have shown that lactobacilli and cocci are abundant (Knarreborg *et al.*, 2002; Van der Wielen *et al.*, 2002; Lu *et al.*, 2003). However the composition of the microbiota, and the abundance of *Clostridia*, varied with different diets (Apajalahti *et al.*, 2001; Knarreborg *et al.*, 2002), probiotics (Netherwood *et al.*, 1999) and monensin (Lu *et al.*, 2006).

These molecular studies have also revealed that the chicken intestine is filled with poorly characterised clostridial species. Apajalahti *et al.* (2001) used G+C% profiling which showed that most of the 16S rDNA sequences detected were not well known bacterial species. These findings were confirmed by Gong *et al.* (2002), Zhu *et al.* (2002) and Lu *et al.* (2003) who determined that many of the 16S rDNA sequences retrieved from a cecal content library exhibited low similarity to known bacterial genera.

4.3. Genetic relationships

The use of growth-promoting antibiotics and probiotics reduces the prevalence of necrotic enteritis. In our studies, these treatments also increased the abundance of *Clostridia* in the ileum (Lu *et al.*, 2006 and unpublished data). In order to investigate the relatedness of the ileal *Clostridia* to characterised strains, we performed a phylogenetic comparison using clostridial 16S rDNA sequences retrieved from GenBank. These were selected based on the *Clostridium* phylogeny proposed by Collins *et al.*, 1994. The majority of the ileal sequences were distantly related to cluster XI, which included *C. lituseburense*, *C. irregularis*, and many environmental clostridia. Many of the novel *Clostridia* detected were most similar to *Fecalobacterium* (formerly *Fusobacterium*) *prausnitzii*, cluster IV, but too dissimilar to be considered members of the *Fecalobacterium* genus. This cluster also includes some pathogenic members but the cluster is very diverse due to discovery of new members associated with intestinal communities. 16S rDNA sequences with high similarity to segmented filamentous bacteria, which are *Clostridia* of uncertain phylogeny, were frequently detected and bacteria related to cluster I, which contains most of the pathogenic *Clostridium* such as *C. tetani*, *C. botulinum*, and *C. perfringens*, were also detected. But only the untreated control group had sequences with high similarity to *C. perfringens* (Lu *et al.*, 2003).

4.4. Novel results

Therefore the chicken intestine contains a novel community of uncharacterised *Clostridia* species. DNA sequencing of the genomes of common cultivable organisms, such as *C. perfringens, Bacteroides thetaiotaomicron,* and *E. coli*, has resulted in a significant knowledge base concerning the ability of bacteria to perform certain functions and express virulence. DNA sequencing of clones acquired from a bacterial community, known as metagenome analysis, allows metabolic and pathogenic predictions about uncultivable bacteria present in the community. These predictions are based on the distribution, characteristics, and identity of genes detected in the community. We used this approach to study the novel community of *Clostridia* present in the chicken intestine. We prepared a metagenome library of bacteria collected from the chicken cecum. Nearly 3000 clones were randomly selected and partial DNA sequences were obtained from each end of the insert. Only a few clones exhibited any DNA similarity to sequences present in GenBank and these were similar to *E. coli*, *Bacteroides*, or *Enterococcus*. While the 16S rDNA library sequences indicated that the metagenome represented *Clostridia*, the G+C content of the metagenome clones was much higher than the majority of the pathogenic *Clostridia*. Pathogenic species of *Clostridium* (such as *C. perfringens, C. chauvoei, C. novii, C. tetani, C. botulinum, C. sordelli*) contain 25-40% G+C while cluster IV (*Fecalobacterium*) tend to contain 50-60% G+C. Most of the metagenome clones contained >50% G+C and many had 60-70%. This indicates that the *Clostridia* sampled by the library were very different from known species. We did not detect virulence determinants in this random screening; therefore in order to evaluate the pathogenic potential of these clostridia we screened the library for expression of lipase and phospholipase activities associated with putative toxin genes. As a control we also screened for sialidase activity, an enzyme frequently produced by mucosal bacteria. We screened approximately 70,000 clones in two different experiments. While we identified several that produced sialidase, no phospholipase or lipase producing clones were detected indicating that these *Clostridia* are not likely to produce α-toxin activity.

Few studies have been published that discuss whether these novel intestinal *Clostridia* may contribute to the health and performance of animals. Umesaki *et al.* (1999) reconstituted gnotobiotic mice with a strain of segmented filamentous bacteria (uncharacterised *Clostridia*) and demonstrated that they induced intestinal development similar to *B. thetaiotaomicron*. We have performed similar studies in day-of-hatch chicks and found that some strains of *Clostridia* enhance intestinal development (unpublished results). Therefore, these species do not contain the necessary array of clostridial virulence determinants and are likely to be nonpathogenic. While behaving as intestinal symbionts, these clostridial communities can also potentially act as a competitively suppressive ecosystem reducing the virulence of *C. perfringens* in the small intestine.

5. Conclusions

It is well accepted that the intestinal microbiota contributes to food animal performance and health but it is not known how specific organisms or populations of organisms affect the host to produce these effects. It is assumed that beneficial effects result when the symbiotic bacteria exclude significant numbers of parasitic bacteria from the intestine. However, it is becoming clear that members of the normal bacterial community may stimulate mucosal immunity (Perdigon *et al.*, 1995; Chin *et al.*, 2000), modulate inflammation (Neish *et al.*, 2000; Verdu *et al.*, 2000), promote enterocyte brush border enzyme activity (Zaouche *et al.*, 2000; Buts *et al.*, 1999; Whitt and Savage, 1988), modulate expression of luminal glycoconjugants (Hooper *et al.*, 1998), and suppress the virulence of pathogens (Craven *et al.*, 1999). We don't yet know specifically which type of community composition is needed to promote good intestinal health and function. Similarly, it is unknown what compositional ratios indicate intestinal disease such as infection or inflammation. However, understanding the development of intestinal bacterial communities is necessary for intelligent design of bacteriotherapies to reduce the level of pathogen carriage by food animals, for antibiotic-free treatment of intestinal diseases, and to improve weight gain and feed conversion.

References

Amann, R.I., Ludwig, W. and Schleiefer, K.H. (1995). Phylogenetic identification and in situ detection of individual microbial cells without cultivation. *Microbiological Reviews* **59:** 143-169.

Apajalahti, J.H.A., Kettunen, A., Bedford, M.R. and Holben, W.E. (2001). Percent G+C profiling accurately reveals diet-related differences in the gastrointestinal microbial community of broiler chickens. Applied and Environmental Microbiology **67:** 5656-5667.

Avaniss-Aghajani, E., Jones, K., Chapman, D. and Brunk, C. (1994). A molecular technique for identification of bacteria using small subunit ribosomal RNA sequences. *BioTechniques* **17:** 144-149.

Barnes, E.M., Mead, G.C., Barnum, D.A. and Harry, E.G. (1972). The intestinal flora of the chicken in the period 2 to 6 weeks of age, with particular reference to the anaerobic bacteria. *British Poultry Science* **13:** 311-326.

Barnes, E.M. (1979). The intestinal microflora of poultry and game birds during life and after storage. *Journal of Applied Bacteriology* **46:** 407-419.

Bry, L., Falk, P.G., Midtvedt, T. and Gordon, J.I. (1996). A model of host-microbial interactions in an open mammalian ecosystem. *Science* **273:** 1380-1383.

Buts, J.P., De Keyser, N., Marandi, S., Hermans, D., Sokal, E.M., Chae, Y.H., Lambotte, L., Chanteux, H. and Tulkens, P.M. (1999). *Saccharomyces boulardii* upgrades cellular adaptation after proximal enterectomy in rats. *Gut* **45:** 89-96.

Chin, J., Turner, B., Barchia, I. and Mullbacher, A. (2000). Immune response to orally consumed antigens and probiotic bacteria. *Immunology and Cell Biology* **78:** 55-66.

Clark, G.C., Briggs, D.C., Karasawa, T., Wang, X., Cole, A.R., Maegawa, T., Jayasekera, P.N., Naylor, C.E., Miller, J., Moss, D.S., Nakamura, S., Basak, A.K. and R.W. Titball (2003). *Clostridium absonum* alpha-toxin: new insights into clostridial phospholipase C substrate binding and specificity. *Journal of Molecular Biology* **333:** 759-769.

Collins, M.D., Lawson, P.A., Willems, A., Cordoba, J.J., Fernandez-Garayzabal, J., Garcia, P., Cai, J., Hippe, H. and Farrow, J.A.E. (1994). The phylogeny of the Genus *Clostridium*: proposal of five new genera and eleven new species combinations. *International Journal of Systematic Bacteriology* **44:** 812-826.

Craven, S.E., Stern, N.J., Cox, N.A., Bailey, J.S. and Berrang. M. (1999). Cecal carriage of *Clostridium perfringens* in broiler chickens given Mucosal Starter Culture. *Avian Diseases* **43:** 484-90.

Decroos, K., Vercauteren, T., Werquin, G. and Verstraete, W. (2004). Repression of *Clostridium* population in young broiler chickens after administration of a probiotic mixture. *Communications in Agric Applied Biological Science* **69:** 5-13.

Drasar, B.S. and Barrow, P.A. (1985). *Intestinal Microbiology*. American Society for Microbiology, Washington, D.C.

Falk, P.G., Hooper, L.V., Midtvedt, T. and Gordon, J.I. (2000). Creating and maintaining the gastrointestinal ecosystem: what we know and need to know from gnotobiology. *Microbiology and Molecular Biology Reviews* **62:** 1157-1170.

Farrelly, V., Rainey, F.A. and Stackebrandt, E. (1995). Effect of genome size and rrn gene copy number on PCR amplification of 16S rRNA genes from a mixture of bacterial species. *Applied and Environmental Microbiology* **61:** 2798-801.

Fukata, T., Hadate, Y., Baba, E. and Arakawa, A. (1991). Influence of bacteria on *Clostridium perfringens* infections in young chickens. *Avian Diseases* **35:** 224-7.

Gong, J., Forster, R.J., Yu, H., Chambers, J.R., Sabour, P.M., Wheatcroft, R. and Chen, S. (2002). Diversity and phylogenetic analysis of bacteria in the mucosa of chicken ceca and comparison with bacteria in the cecal lumen. *FEMS Microbiology Letters* **208:** 1-7.

Gordon, H. A. and Pesti, L. (1971). The gnotobiotic animal as a tool in the study of host microbial relationships. *Bacteriological Reviews* **35:** 390-429.

Hofacre, C.L., Froyman, R., Gautrias, B., George, B., Goodwin, M.A. and Brown, J. (1998a). Use of Aviguard and other intestinal bioproducts in experimental *Clostridium perfringens*-associated necrotizing enteritis in broiler chickens. *Avian Diseases* **42:** 579-584.

Hofacre, C.L., Froyman, R., George, B., Goodwin, M.A. and Brown, J. (1998b). Use of Aviguard, virginiamycin, or bacitracin MD against *Clostridium perfringens*-associated necrotizing enteritis. *Journal of Applied Poultry Research* **7:** 412-418.

Hooper, L.V., Bry, L., Falk, P.G. and Gordon, J.I. (1998). Host-microbial symbiosis in the mammalian intestine: exploring an internal ecosystem. *Bioessays* **20:** 336-343.

Karasawa, T., Wang, X., Maegawa, T., Michiwa, Y., Kita, H., Miwa, K. and Nakamura, S. (2003). *Clostridium sordellii* phospholipase C: gene cloning and comparison of enzymatic and biological activities with those of *Clostridium perfringens* and *Clostridium bifermentans* phospholipase C. *Infection and Immunity* **71:** 641-646.

Kaldhusdal, M., Schneitz, C., Hofshagen, M. and Skjerve, E. (2001). Reduced incidence of *Clostridium perfringens*-associated lesions and improved performance in broiler chickens treated with normal intestinal bacteria from adult fowl. *Avian Diseases* **45:** 149-156.

Kitts, C.L. (2001). Terminal restriction fragment patterns: a tool for comparing microbial communities and assessing community dynamics. *Current Issues in Intestinal Microbiology* **2:** 17-25.

Knarreborg, A., Simon, M.A., Engberg, R.M., Jensen, B.B. and Tannock, G.W. (2002). Effects of dietary fat source and subtherapeutic levels of antibiotic on the bacterial community in the ileum of broiler chickens at various ages. *Applied and Environmental Microbiology* **68:** 5918-5924.

Lu, J., Idris, U., Harmon, B., Hofacre, C., Maurer, J.J. and Lee, M.D. (2003). Diversity and succession of the intestinal bacterial community of the maturing broiler chicken. *Applied and Environmental Microbiology* **69:** 6816-6824.

Lu, J., Hofacre, C. and Lee, M.D. (2006). Emerging Technologies in Microbial Ecology Aid in Understanding the Complex Disease Necrotic Enteritis. *Journal of Applied Poultry Research* **15:** 145-153.

Madden, J.A.J. and Hunter, J.O. (2002). A review of the role of the gut microflora in irritable bowel syndrome and the effects of probiotics. *British Journal of Nutrition* **88:** S67-S72.

Mead, G.C. (1989). Microbes of the avian cecum: types present and substrates utilized. *Journal of Experimental Zoology. Supplement* **3:** 48-54.

Neish, A.S., Gewitz, A.T., Zeng, H., Young, A.N., Hobert, M., Karmali, V., Rao, A.S., and Madara, J.L. (2000). Prokaryotes regulate epithelial responses by inhibition of IκB-α ubiquitination. *Science* **289:** 1560-1563.

Neish, A.S. (2002). The gut microflora and intestinal epithelial cells: a continuing dialogue. *Microbes and Infection* **4:** 309-317.

Netherwood, T., Gilbert, H.J., Parker, D.S. and O'Donnell, A.G. (1999). Probiotics shown to change bacterial community structure in the avian gastrointestinal tract. *Applied and Environmental Microbiology* **65:** 5134-5138.

Ohtani, K., Hayashi, H. and Shimizu, T. (2002). The luxS gene is involved in cell-cell signalling for toxin production in *Clostridium perfringens. Molecular Microbiology* **44:** 171-179.

Parish, W.E. (1961). Necrotic enteritis in the fowl. *Journal of Comparative Pathology* **74:** 377-393.

Perdigon, G., Alvarez, S., Rachid, M., Aguero, G. and Gobbato, N. (1995). Immune system stimulation by probiotics. *Journal of Dairy Science* **78:** 1597-1606.

Petit, L., Gibert, M. and Popoff, M.R. (1999). *Clostridium perfringens*: toxinotype and genotype. *Trends in Microbiology* **7:** 104-110.

Rafter, J. (2002). Lactic acid bacteria and cancer: mechanistic perspective. *British Journal of Nutrition* **88:** S67-S72.

Rood, J.I. (1998). Virulence genes of *Clostridium perfringens. Annual Review of Microbiology* **52:** 333-360.

Salanitro, J.P., Fairchilds, I.G. and Zgornicki, Y.D. (1974). Isolation, culture characteristics, and identification of anaerobic bacteria from the chicken cecum. *Applied Microbiology* **27:** 678-687.

Schaedler, R.W., Dubos, R. and Costello, R. (1965). Association of germfree mice with bacteria isolated from normal mice. *Journal of Experimental Medicine* **122:** 77-82.

Schaller, D. (1998). Necrotic enteritis in poultry production - the Norwegian experience. *Proceedings of European Poultry Symposium*, Bayer AG, Cascais, Portugal. pp. 37-42.

Simpson, J.M., McCracken, V.J., White, B.A., Gaskins, H.R. and Mackie, R.I. (1999). Application of denaturant gradient gel electrophoresis for the analysis of the porcine gastrointestinal microbiota. *Journal of Microbiological Methods* **36:** 167-179.

Staley, J.T. and Konopka, A. (1985). Measurement of in situ activites of nonphotosynthetic microorganisms in aquatic and terrestrial habitats. *Annual Review of Microbiology* **39:** 321-346.

Stappenbeck, T.S., Hooper, L.V., Manchester, J.K., Wong, M.H. and Gordon, J.I. (2002). Laser capture microdissection of mouse intestine: characterizing mRNA and protein expression, and profiling intermediary metabolism in specified cell populations. *Methods in Enzymology* **356:** 167-196.

Suau, A., Bonnet, R., Sutren, M., Godon, J., Gibson, G.R., Collins, M.D. and Dore, J. (1999). Direct analysis of gene encoding 16S rRNA from complex communities reveals many novel molecular species within the human gut. *Applied and Environmental Microbiology* **65:** 4799-4807.

Suzuki, M.T. and Giovannoni, S.J. (1996). Bias caused by template annealing in the amplification of mixtures of 16S rRNA genes by PCR. *Applied and Environmental Microbiology* **62:** 625-630.

Umesaki, Y., Setoyama, H., Matsumoto, S., Imaoka A. and Itoh, K. (1999). Differential Roles of Segmented Filamentous Bacteria and Clostridia in Development of the Intestinal Immune System. *Infection and Immunity* **67:** 3504-3511.

Van der Wielen, P.W., Keuzenkamp, D.A., Lipman, L.J., van Knapen, F. and Biesterveld, S. (2002). Spatial and temporal variation of the intestinal bacterial community in commercially raised broiler chickens during growth. *Microbial Ecology* **44:** 286-293.

Van Immerseel, F., De Buck, J., Pasmans, F., Huyghebaert, G., Haesebrouck, F. and Ducatelle, R. (2004). *Clostridium perfringens* in poultry: an emerging threat for animal and public health. *Avian Pathology* **33:** 537-549.

Verdu, E.F., Bercik, P., Cukrowska, B., Farre-Castany, M.A., Bouzourene, H., Saraga, E., Blum, A.L., Corthesy-Theulaz, I., Tlaskalova-Hogenova, H. and Michetti, P. (2000). Oral administration of antigens from intestinal flora anaerobic bacteria reduces the severity of experimental acute colitis in BALB/c mice. *Clinical and Experimental Immunology* **120:** 46-50.

Wages, D.P. and Opengart, K. (2003). Necrotic Enteritis. *In:* Y.M. Saif (Ed.), Diseases of Poultry, 11th Ed. Iowa State University Press, Ames, Iowa. pp. 781-785.

Whitt, D.D. and Savage, D.C. (1988). Influence of indigenous microbiota on activities of alkaline phosphatase, phosphodiesterase I, and thymidine kinase in mouse enterocytes. *Applied and Environmental Microbiology* **54:** 2405-2410.

Williams, R.B. (2005). Intercurrent coccidiosis and necrotic enteritis of chickens: rational, integrated disease management by maintenance of gut integrity. *Avian Pathology* **34:** 159-180.

Xu J. and Gordon, J.I. (2003). Inaugural Article: Honor thy symbionts. *Proceedings of the National Academy of Science USA* **100:** 10452-10459.

Zaouche, A., Loukil, C., De Lagausie, P., Peuchmaur, M., Macry, J., Fitoussi, F., Bernasconi, P., Bingen, E. and Cezard, J.P. (2000). Effects of oral *Saccharomyces boulardii* on bacterial overgrowth, translocation, and intestinal adaptation after small-bowel resection in rats. *Scandinavian Journal of Gastroenterology* **35:** 160-165.

Zhu, X.Y., Zhong, T., Pandya, Y. and Joerger, R. D. (2002). 16S rRNA-based analysis of microbiota from the cecum of broiler chickens. *Applied and Environmental Microbiology* **68:** 124-137.

Zoetendal, E.G., Akkermans, A.D.L. and de Vos, W.M. (1998). Temperature gradient gel electrophoresis analysis of 16S rRNA from human fecal samples reveals stable and host-specific communities of active bacterial. *Applied and Environmental Microbiology* **64:** 3854-3854.

Coccidiosis control: yesterday, today and tomorrow

Hafez Mohamed Hafez
Institute of Poultry Diseases, Faculty of Veterinary Medicine, Free University Berlin, Königsweg 63, 14163 Berlin, Germany

1. Introduction

Coccidiosis is the major parasitic disease of poultry with substantial economic losses due to malabsorption, reduced feed conversion, reduced weight gain and increased mortality. In addition, the use of anticoccidial drugs and /or vaccines for treatment and prevention, contributes a major production cost.

1.1. Aetiology

Coccidia are protozoa which have the ability to multiply rapidly inside cells lining the intestine or caeca. The species of coccidia that are infective to poultry belong to the *Eimeria* genus. Many of these species can infect poultry and there is no cross-immunity between them. Most infestations under field conditions are mixed but one species will be dominant. *Eimeria* have a self-limiting life cycle and are characterised by a high tissue and host specificity.

The *Eimeria* cycle includes two distinct phases; (a) the internal phase (schizogony + gamogony) in which the parasite multiplies in different parts of the intestinal tract and the oocysts are excreted in the faeces (The part of the intestinal tract and the total duration of the internal phase of the cycle is dependant on species), (b) the external phase (sporogony) during which the oocyst must undergo a final process called sporulation before they are again infective. Sporulation requires warmth (25-30 °C), moisture and oxygen (Levine, 1982).

Seven species of *Eimeria* are known to infect chickens and they show a wide variation in their pathogenicity (Table 1). In addition, two further species have been described, namely *E. hagani* and *E. mivati*, but further studies on the importance of these species are needed (Conway and McKenzie, 2007).

In turkeys seven species of *Eimeria* have been reported (Table 2), however *E. innocua and E subrotunda* are considered non-pathogenic (Trees, 1990, McDougald, 2003).

Table 1. Some characteristics of important Eimeria spp. infecting chickens.

Host	Eimeria	Location	Pathogenicity[1]
Chickens	*E. acervulina*	duodenum, jejunum	++
	E. brunetti	ileum, rectum	+++
	E. maxima	duodenum, jejunum, ileum	++
	E. mitis	duodenum, jejunum	+
	E. necatrix	jejunum, caeca	+++
	E. praecox	duodenum, jejunum	+
	E. tenella	caeca	+++

[1]- non-pathogenic; + mildly pathogenic; ++ moderately pathogenic; +++ highly pathogenic.

Table 2. Some characteristics of important Eimeria spp. infecting turkeys.

Host	Eimeria	Location	Pathogenicity[1]
Turkeys	*E. adenoeides*	caecum	+++
	E. dispersa	duodenum, jejunum	+
	E. gallopavonis	rectum	++
	E innocua	duodenum, jejunum	-
	E. meleagridis	caecum	+
	E. meleagrimitis	duodenum, jejunum	+++
	E. subrotunda	duodenum, jejunum	-

[1]- non-pathogenic; + mildly pathogenic; ++ moderately pathogenic; +++ highly pathogenic.

Geese are parasitised by two species; *Eimeria truncata* (unusually this is found in the kidney) and *Eimeria anseris.* A large number of specific coccidia have been also reported in ducks, but the validity of some of them is still not clear. The most pathogenic coccidial infection of ducks is *Tyzzeria perniciosa,* which causes haemorrhagic enteritis in ducklings less than 7 weeks of age (Trees, 1990, McDougald, 2003).

1.2. Transmission

The oocysts are extraordinary resistant to environmental stress and disinfectants, remaining viable in the litter for many months. Temperatures above 56 °C and below 0 °C are lethal but it seems to be impossible to decontaminate a previously contaminated poultry house or environment. Sporulated oocysts can be spread mechanically by wild birds, insects or rodents and via contaminated boots, clothing, equipment or dust. Direct oral transmission is the natural route of infection (McDougald, 2003).

1.3. Clinical signs and lesions

Several *Eimeria* species are able to cause clinical signs in infected and unprotected birds; however subclinical infections are frequently seen. These are often underestimated but mostly result in impaired feed conversion and reduced weight gain.

Coccidiosis generally occurs more frequently during the warmer months of the year (Smith, 1995). Young birds are more susceptible and more readily display signs of disease, whereas older chickens are relatively resistant as a result of prior infection.

The severity of an infection depends on the age of birds, *Eimeria* species, number of sporulated oocysts ingested, immune status of the flock and environmental management.

Infected birds tend to huddle together, have ruffled feathers and show signs of depression. The birds consume less feed and water, and droppings are watery to whitish or bloody. This results in dehydration and poor weight gain as well as mortalities.

The lesions of coccidiosis depend on the degree of inflammation and damage to the intestinal tract. They include thickness of the intestinal wall, mucoid to blood-tinged exudates, petechial haemorrhages, necrosis, haemorrhagic enteritis and mucous profuse bleeding in the caeca.

The tissue damage in the intestinal tract may allow secondary colonisation by various bacteria, such as *Clostridium perfringens* (Helmbolt and Bryant, 1971), or *Salmonella Typhimurium* (Arakawa *et al.*, 1981, Baba *et al.*, 1982). Infestation with *E. tenella* also increases the severity of *Histomonas meleagridis* infection in chickens (McDougald and Hu, 2001).

1.4. Diagnosis

Coccidiosis is often extremely difficult to diagnose and can only be done in the laboratory (Conway and McKenzie, 2007), by counting coccidia per gram of faeces and/or examining the intestinal tract to determine the lesion scores, as described by Johnson and Reid (1970). The estimation of the lesion scores is difficult in turkeys (Irion, 1999). Since it is common for healthy birds to possess some coccidia, consideration of flock history and lesion score must be carefully evaluated before making a diagnosis or treatment recommendations.

Intestinal coccidiosis may be confused with necrotic enteritis, haemorrhagic enteritis, or other enteric diseases. Caecal coccidiosis may be confused with histomoniasis and salmonellosis due to their similar lesions (Hafez, 1997).

2. Prevention and control: yesterday, today and tomorrow

In the past it has been realised that eradication of coccidia is not realistic and hygienic measures alone are not able to prevent infections. However, if an outbreak of coccidiosis occurs, treatment via the drinking water should start as soon as possible. The most commonly used drugs are sulphonamides, amprolium and toltrazuril. Today the prevention and control of coccidiosis is based on chemotherapy, using anticoccidial drugs and /or vaccines along with hygienic measures and improved farm management.

2.1. Anticoccidial drugs

According to Shirley and Chapman (2005) the most significant study that had the greatest impact on control of coccidiosis was that of Delaplane *et al.* (1947) which showed that the administration of low concentrations of sulphaquinoxaline in the feed effectively controlled the disease.

The rapid development of the broiler industry in the 1950s required the urgent availability of anticoccidial drugs. This soon led to intensive activities by several companies to produce a range of chemical products that were effective in the control coccidiosis. However, these products also prevented treated birds from building up any natural immunity and they were not effective enough to kill all exposed coccidia. The result was that the surviving coccidia quickly became resistant to the products and severe outbreaks of the disease occurred. According to Chapman (1994a) nicarbazin was introduced in 1955 to the USA and was extensively used in broiler production. In the 1970s several other highly efficacious synthetic drugs were introduced but due to the rapid development of drug resistance, they were withdrawn shortly afterwards. The development of resistance was documented for these anticoccidial chemical drugs (Jeffers, 1974a,b; McDougald *et al.*,1986). It is likely that resistance has developed to more recent anticoccidial drugs but this has not been investigated and may have gone unrecorded (Chapman, 2005).

A major enhancement in coccidiosis control occurred in the 1970s with the introduction of monensin as the first ionophore coccidiostat. Introduction of ionophores changed the ability to control coccidiosis – an impact that remains to this day (Shirley and Chapman, 2005). The effectiveness of ionophore coccidiostats lies in the fact that whilst they kill the majority of the invading parasites, they permit a small leakage of coccidia enabling a degree of host immunity to develop. Resistance to ionophores develops very slowly and there is more of a tendency to increased levels of tolerance. Chapman and Hacker (1994) as well as Mathis (1999) observed a marginal to poor effect of different ionophores to several *Eimeria sp.*

Since the 1970s, coccidiostats have been regulated under the Feed Additives Directive 524/70/EEC (EEC, 1970, 2004), which has now been replaced by Regulation No 1831/2003/ EC (EC, 2003, 2007). As such, they have not been subject to veterinary prescription status, since they are required routinely in the feed of commercial broilers and turkeys.

Currently several types of anticcocidial drugs are available including synthetic compounds (chemicals), quinalone and certain ionophore antibiotics (Table 3). In recent years, however, few new drugs have been introduced. All types of drug used for coccidiosis control are unique; in their mode of action, the way in which parasites are killed or arrested, and the effects of the drug on the growth and performance of the bird. Very few drugs are equally efficacious against all *Eimeria* species (McDougald, 2003).

The efficiency of anticoccidial agents can be reduced by drug resistance and management programmes are designed to prevent this developing, which results in better gut health and feed utilisation by birds. Using a drug rotation, with constant monitoring of the oocysts in the faeces and in the litter, or shuttle

Table 3. Some anticoccidial drugs used for prevention in chickens and turkeys in the EU.

Generic name	Brand name (Manufacturer)	Category of animals	Max. age (weeks)	Conc. (ppm)		Withdrawal time (days)
				Min.	Max.	
Diclazuril	Clinacox (Janssen)	Broiler	-	1	1	5
		Pullets	16	1	1	
		Turkey	12	1	1	
Decoquinate	Deccox (Alpharma)	Broiler	-	30	50	3
Halofuginone	Stenorol (Huvepharma)	Broiler	-	2	3	5
		Pullets	16	2	3	
		Turkey	12	2	3	
Lasalocid sodium	Avatec (Alpharma)	Broiler	-	75	125	5
		Pullets	16	75	125	
		Turkey	12	90	125	
Maduramicin ammonium	Cygro (Alpharma)	Broiler	-	5	5	5
		Turkey	16	5	5	
Monensin sodium	Elancoban (Elanco)	Broiler	-	100	125	3
		Pullets	16	100	125	
		Turkey	16	60	100	
Monensin sodium	Coxidin (Huvepharma)	Broiler	-	100	125	3
		Turkey	16	90	100	
Narasin	Monteban (Elanco)	Broiler	-	70	70	1
Narasin/ Nicarbazin	Maxiban (Elanco)	Broiler	-	80	100	5
Robenidine HCl	Cycostat (Alpharma)	Broiler	-	30	36	5
		Turkey	-	30	36	
Salinomycin sodium	Sacox (Huvepharma)	Broiler	-	60	70	1
		Pullets	12	50	50	
Salinomycin sodium	Salinomax (Alpharma)	Broiler	-	50	70	1
Semduramicin	Aviax (Forum)	Broiler	-	20	25	5

programme (ionophore/ chemical) seems to be of great value. Rotation involves changing the product used every 4–6 months. The alternative to a rotation programme is a continuous program where the same products are used until a problem develops or until a new product is introduced on the market. Rotations

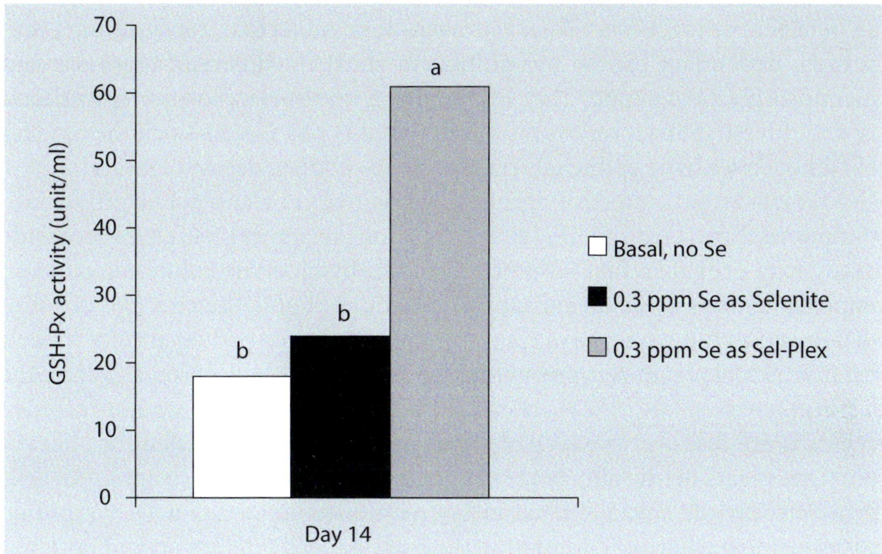

Figure 1. Effect of maternal Se source on plasma GSH-Px activity of broiler chicks (Ao et al., *2006).*

N-linked glycans with a core structure of Man $_{10\text{-}14}$ GlcNAc2-Asn (Lipke and Ovalle, 1998). These structures are very similar to mannose-rich N-glycan chains that are associated with cell surface structures found on mammalian cells. Outer chains present on yeast mannoproteins consist of from 50 to 200 additional α-linked mannose units, with a long α-1,6-linked backbone decorated with short α-1,2 and α-1,3-linked side chains.

An extremely large set of empirical observations have clearly established that the use of mannan-rich cell wall fractions in animal feeding strategies can have beneficial effects on animal health and productivity. While it is not always clear how these functional carbohydrate fractions can influence animal physiology, the use of glycomics and applied animal studies has made it possible to describe some of the complex primary activities of the yeast cell wall product, Bio-Mos.

The best characterised activity of Bio-Mos is associated with its ability to agglutinate or aggregate bacterial cells containing Type 1 fimbriae. In the gastrointestinal tract, lectins (carbohydrate-binding proteins) on bacterial cells bind to complementary carbohydrates on animal epithelial cell surfaces. This process is critical to the initiation of bacterial colonisation and any associated pathogenesis. This pathogen-host molecular recognition event is often dependent on the recognition of short oligomers of mannose and mannose glycoconjugates that extend from the surface of the epithelium. Several investigators have hypothesised that it is possible to block the binding of pathogen with the epithelial receptor site by adding 'decoy oligosaccharides' also known as 'anti-infective' agents based on mannose and polymannose into the animal diets (Oyofo *et al.*, 1989a). As result, an appropriate oligosaccharide decoy may provide a first level of protection by blocking colonisation. More importantly, this mechanistic approach does not apply the selective pressure that results in the evolution of resistance in the targeted pathogen since there is environmental parameters preventing the growth of organisms that produce the lectin containing fimbriea. As result, the beneficial effect of these anti-infective agents is not lost over time. Oyofo and coworkers (1989b) tested the effect of different sugars on the adherence of *Salmonella typhimurium* to epithelial cells from one-day-old chicks and found that mannose and methyl-α-D-mannoside were the most efficient in inhibiting the bacterial/cell interaction and bacterial adherence. They reported that mannose addition to *in vitro* systems decreased the number of adherent bacterial cells to a defined intestinal surface by more than 90% when compared to a control with no carbohydrate added. This confirmed earlier *in vitro* studies that indicated differences exist in the ability of different mannose-based sugars to block pathogen attachment. Firon and coworkers (1985) demonstrated that compounds containing both α-1,3 and α-1,6 branched mannan (as found in the outer cell wall of *S. cerevisiae*) had approximately 37.5 times greater ability to prevent the adsorption of *E. coli* then did D-mannose. In these studies, the specific structure of the mannan product clearly defined its functional properties. Since the cost of using purified mannose sugars or mannoligosaccharides for large scale use as anti-infective activities is cost prohibitive, the use of mannose containing complex like those naturally found in yeast cell wall preparations are attractive for use in strategies for controlling certain types of bacterial infections in the gastrointestinal tract. In the last decade, a number of studies have clearly demonstrated that the strategic use of yeast cell wall fractions can be used to reduce the concentrations of pathogenic bacteria in the gastrointestinal tract (Spring *et al.*, 2000)

Probably one of the most important roles for Bio-Mos appears to be related to its ability to modify the morphology and structure of the intestinal mucosa. This is a role that has only recently been recognised. However, it is not clear whether this is a direct effect or an indirect effect resulting from changes in the gastrointestinal microbial ecology. Early studies at Oregon State University demonstrated a reduction in crypt depth of turkey poults fed diets containing

0.1% Bio-Mos for eight weeks (Savage *et al.*, 1997). These changes in crypt depth were correlated to a statistically significant increase in growth rate through eight weeks of age, suggesting an inverse correlation between the parameters measured. Other studies have shown that inclusion of yeast cell wall at 0.2% in broiler diets aided in intestinal development with an increase in villus height during the first seven days of life and could be positively correlated with an improved body weight gain over the entire production period (Santin *et al.*, 2001). Another detailed study evaluated the response of the intestinal mucosa of broiler chickens when Bio-Mos was included in sorghum/lupin-based diets at 0.0, 1.0, 3.0 or 5.0g/kg diet (Iji *et al.*, 2003). Supplementation with the highest level of Bio-Mos resulted in longer ($P<0.01$) jejunal villi. The RNA content of the ileal mucosal homogenate was significantly greater ($P<0.05$) in chicks receiving 3.0 and 5.0g Bio-Mos/kg diet than in other groups. The protein/RNA and RNA/DNA ratios in ileal homogenates were significantly ($P<0.01$) influenced by the presence of Bio-Mos in the diet. This was not translated into increased mucosal growth or differences in digestive enzyme activities in the ileum. However, with Bio-Mos inclusion in the diet, there were significantly greater specific activities of maltase ($P<0.01$), leucine aminopeptidase ($P<0.05$) and alkaline phosphatase ($P<0.001$) in the jejunum. Uni and Smirov (2006) investigated the possibility that the addition of Bio-Mos to a broiler diet may have an effect on both mucin biosynthesis and secretion in the small intestine. The results of their study showed that MOS had a stimulating effect on the mucin dynamic. Feeding Bio-Mos at 2g/kg increased the size of goblet cell, mucin production and the mucus thickness layers in comparison to the negative control diet and a diet containing an antimicrobial growth promotant. Interestingly, inclusion of Bio-Mos in the diet increased the mRNA expression of the MUC 2 gene as determined by semi-quantitative RT-PCR (Figure 2). The authors hypothesise that Bio-Mos may interact with cell membrane lectins, which can regulate cell growth and survival by interacting with cytoplasmic and nuclear proteins thereby affecting intracellular signaling pathways. These studies suggest that mannanoligosaccharides, specifically Bio-Mos, can be related to improved growth efficiencies through a mechanism that alters the structural and functional activities of the tissues. This may truly be an unrecognised role for functional carbohydrates in nutrition and may provide new tools for enhancing animal performance in modern animal production systems.

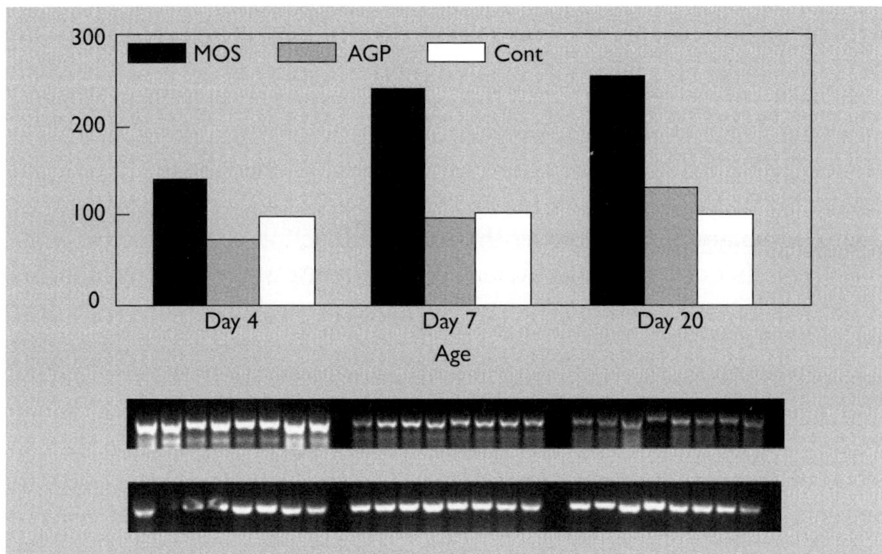

Figure 2. Mucin mRNA expression in the different treatments. Top panel: Changes in Mucin mRNA expression. Bottom panel: Representative picture of intestinal Mucin mRNA and 18S rRNA amplification at day 28 in the jejunum.

8. Selenium supplementation: effects on poultry performance and wellbeing

Ever since its discovery in the early 1800s, selenium has presented a nutritional suconundrum because of its dual status as a potentially toxic but highly essential trace element. However, research carried out over the past decade has resulted in recognition of organic selenium supplementation as a key element in improving animal nutrition, health and wellbeing. Research has clearly shown that dietary intervention with organic selenium can result in significantly enhanced production and health in all species. Some of the most striking findings are that nutritional supplementation with organic selenium resulted in; increased live young per animal, stimulation of immune function, overall improvements in animal health and enhanced shelf life of meat and eggs (Table 1).

Whilst these observations can be attributed to general enhancements in cellular antioxidant status and amelioration of the effects of oxidative stress, the exact mechanisms by which these effects are mediated are still largely unclear. Recently, we have used transcriptomics to determine the mechanisms

Table 1. Disease states and health benefits associated with selenium (adapted from McCartney, 2006).

Animal disease states associated with low selenium status	Health and product quality benefits from selenium supplementation
Pancreatic atrophy in chicks	Improved anti-oxidant defence systems, resulting in better resistance against disease
Exudative diathesis - chicks	Enhanced immune responses
Encephalomalacia - chicks	Superior resistance to viral diseases
Muscular dystrophy - chicks	Maintenance of thyroid function
Impaired feathering - poultry	Improved fertility
Reduced egg production	Longer productive life in breeding animals
Increased dead-in-shell chicks	Enhanced Se content of meat and eggs
Poor egg hatchability	Improved meat colour, reduced drip loss
Low chick weights at hatching	Enhanced product freshness, better keeping quality
Suboptimal immunocompetence	
Reproductive failure and infertility - all species	

responsible for these effects. This approach enabled the effects of selenium on gene expression to be demonstrated for the first time and will eventually enable the adoption of a finely directed approach to dietary intervention.

9. Nutrigenomics and organic selenium supplementation

In order to fully appreciate the benefits of organic selenium supplementation, genotypic changes, which are in part responsible for the observed physical changes, must be considered. With this in mind, Alltech initiated a nutrigenomics research programme to study the effects of organic selenium supplementation at the molecular level. Using microarray technologies, a specific branch of nutrigenomics, transcriptomics, was utilised to determine how nutritional exposure to organic selenium affects gene expression in a tissue-specific fashion (Dawson, 2006). The results of this work have reinforced our thinking on the health benefits to be derived from selenium addition to the diet. However, it should be noted that it is only through applying a systems biology approach to the interpretation of experimental data derived from transcriptomics work, that we will be able to fully understand and explain the health benefits of dietary intervention and supplementation. This is an area that is currently being pursued to enable full understanding of transcriptomics results that have been derived from model-animal studies.

To date, this transcriptomics-based approach has compared the expression responses of genes to selenium supplementation with organic Sel-Plex® and inorganic selenite supplementation of poultry diets in a tissue-specific fashion.

Some notable points from this work are as follows:
- Selenium supplementation altered the expression of over 1300 different genes in intestinal tissue and over 5100 genes in oviduct tissue
- Expression of both beneficial and detrimental genes was altered,
- Not all forms of selenium gave the same response,
- More beneficial genes were expressed when Sel-Plex® was added to the diet and expression of stress-associated genes was depressed,
- Gene-expression patterns were consistent with lower levels of oxidative stress in tissues from trial subjects fed Sel-Plex®.

One of the greatest benefits of improved selenium status is the overall reduction in cellular oxidative stress. In the aforementioned studies, supplementation with Sel-Plex® was shown to induce a statistically significant reduction in the expression of stress-response genes through both an increase in the selenium status of the cell and an increase in the expression of genes encoding antioxidant proteins; genes encoding the key antioxidant proteins, GSH-Px 1 and Thioredoxin reductase, were upregulated. The effect of selenium supplementation on the expression levels of GSH-Px 4 is illustrated in Figure 3.

Other genes that were upregulated after selenium addition included Thioredoxin 2 and Iodothyronine deiodinase, both of which play key roles in fertility. Transcript levels of the genes encoding both these proteins, which are involved in implantation and embryonic development, were also significantly increased.

Additional studies examined the expression of genes in tissues such as the cerebral cortex, intestine, liver and skeletal muscle. One of the main genes studied encoded the GADD45β (growth arrest and DNA damage-inducible) gene. This gene is involved in the regulation of cell cycle and apoptosis (programmed cell death) and has been shown to be induced in response to oxidative stress and, in particular, in response to DNA damage. Expression of this gene is now

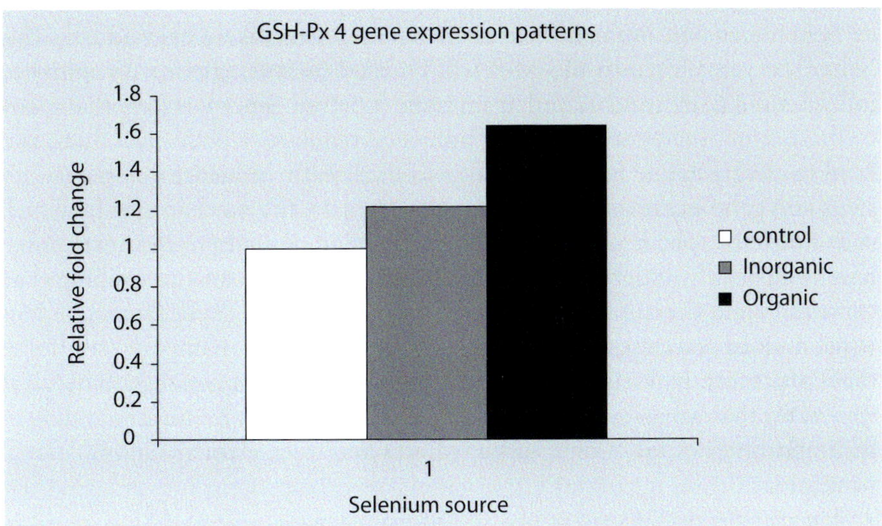

Figure 3. Avian duodenal GSH-Px 4 gene expression patterns in response to selenium supplementation.

recognised as an excellent marker for these stressors. The studies found that GADD45β expression levels were significantly decreased across all tissues by Sel-Plex® treatment but not by treatment with other forms of selenium. This indicates lower endogenous oxidative stress and DNA damage throughout the entire animal and demonstrates the superiority of organic selenium in the form of Sel-Plex® over other selenium sources. The expression of another DNA damage checkpoint gene, MAPK p38α was also significantly decreased in response to organic supplementation with Sel-Plex, again reinforcing the benefits of dietary intervention with selenium.

10. Future of nutrigenomics in animal production

There is a growing recognition that trace elements and functional carbohydrates play a vital role in cellular metabolism, protein structure and function, cell-to-cell communication and host immunity. An understanding of the role of these nutrients will provide new tools for beneficially manipulating metabolism in avian species. In modern poultry production systems, it is becoming increasingly apparent that alternative approaches to conventional antibiotic therapy are required to control infectious diseases and improving the nutrition of poultry species. In the future, nutrigenomics studies using functional carbohydrates and organic trace elements may very likely help address this issue. The yeast fraction Bio-Mos will be used increasingly for it's ability to influence gut health and modulate immune function. Since it is clear that many of these functional carbohydrates influence regulatory pathways, there is a need to clearly define how such compounds directly influence key regulatory steps and gene expression in animal cells. To date, the mechanisms by which such nutrients specifically regulate the expression of genes in the host animal have been poorly understood. The complexity of mechanisms controlling gene expression and the difficulties associated with identifying specific metabolites which induce responses in intestinal epithelium cells has hampered studies of these processes. By focusing on gene expression and functional genomics it is very likely that we will soon be able to gain a more definitive understanding of the importance of functional carbohydrates and trace elements in nutritional strategies.

It is also evident that organic selenium supplementation elicits changes at the molecular level, which increase anti-oxidant status in a whole-body fashion. Nutrigenomics studies have shown that such changes are a consequence of enhancement of selenium status through a reduction in the expression levels of genes encoding oxidative-stress response proteins and an increase in the expression of genes encoding anti-oxidant proteins. We also expect that other positive responses to selenium supplementation such as maternal transfer of selenium, increased selenium concentration in eggs and meat, and a general reduction in illness all stem from effects at the molecular level.

11. Conclusions

Further advances in the fields of nutrigenomics, proteomics and metabolomics will enable researchers to ask key questions about diet and its effects on an organism. By focusing on gene expression and functional genomics, it is very likely that we will soon be able to gain a more definitive understanding of the importance of dietary intervention in nutritional strategies. Whilst still in its infancy, this new scientific frontier will revolutionise our thinking about how dietary supplementation can have such dramatic and beneficial responses on whole body health.

References

Ao, T., Cantor, A.H., Power, R.A., Pierce, J.L., Pescatore, A.J. and Ford, M.J. (2006). Maternal dietary Sel-Plex® (Selenium Yeast) supplementation increases tissue and glutathione peroxidase activity of broiler chicks. *Poultry Science Poscal* **85** (Supplement 1): 112.

Burt, D.W. (2002). Applications of biotechnology in the poultry industry. *Worlds Poultry Science Journal* **58:** 5-13.

Dawson, K.A. (2006). Functional genomics: promising new tools relating nutrition to reproductive responses in cattle. In: *Biotechnology in the Feed Industry, Proceedings of Alltech's 22nd Annual Symposium*, pp. 341-351. (eds. T.P. Lyons and K.A. Jacques). Nottingham University Press, Nottingham, UK.

Firon, N., Duksin, D. and Sharon, N. (1985) Mannose-specific adherence of Escherichia coli To bhk cells that differ in their glycosylation patterns. *FEMS Microbiology Letters* **27**: 161-165.

International Chicken Genome Sequencing Consortium. (2004).Sequence and comparative analysis of the chicken genome provide unique perspectives on vertebrate evolution. *Nature* **432**: 695-716.

International Chicken Polymorphism Map Consortium. (2004). A genetic variation map for chicken with 2.8 million single-nucleotide polymorphisms *Nature* **432**: 717-722.

Iji, P.A., Khumalo, K., Slippers, S. and Gous, R.M. (2003). Intestinal function and body growth of broiler chickens on diets based on maize dried at different temperatures and supplemented with a microbial enzyme. *Reproduction Nutrition Development* **43**: p. 77-90.

Lipke, P.N. and Ovalle, R. (1998). Cell wall architecture in yeast: New structure and new challenges. *Journal of Bacteriology* **180**: 3735-3740.

McCartney, E. (2006). Selenium: An essential nutrient for animals and humans. *World poultry* **2**: 16–18.

Moody, D.E. (2001). Genomic techniques: an overview of methods for the study of gene expression. *Journal of Animal Science* **79** (Suppl. E), E128-E135.

Muller, M. and Kersten, S. (2003). Nutrigenomics: goals and strategies. *Nature Reviews* **4**: 315–322.

Oyofo, B.A., Droleskey, R.E., Norman, J.O., Mollenhauer, H.H., Ziprin, R.L., Corrier, D.E. and Deloach, J.R. (1989a). Inhibition by mannose of in vitro colonization of chicken small intestine by *Salmonella typhimurium. Poultry Science* **68**: 1351-1356.

Oyofo, B.A., Deloach, J.R., Corrier, D.E., Norman, J.O., Ziprin, R.L. and Mollenhauer, H.H. (1989b). Effect of carbohydrates on *Salmonella typhimurium* colonization in broiler chickens. *Avian Diseases* **33**: 531-534.

Savage, T.F., Cotter, P.F. and Zakrzewska, E.I. (1996). The effect of feeding mannanoligosaccharide on immunoglobulins, plasma IgG and bile IgA, of Wrolsted MW male turkeys. *Poultry Science* **75** (Suppl 1): 143.

Savage, T.F., Zakrzewska, E.I. and Andreasen, J.R. (1997) The effects of feeding mannan oligosaccharide supplemented diets to poults on performance and the morphology of the small intestine. *Poultry Science* **76** (Suppl 1): 139.

Santin, E., Maiorka, A., Macari, M., Grecco, M., Sanchez, J.C., Okada, T.M. and Myasaka, A.M. (2001). Performance and intestinal mucosa development of broiler chickens fed diets containing Saccharomyces cerevisiae cell wall. *Journal of Applied Poultry Research* **10**: 236-244.

Spring, P., Wenk, C., Dawson, K.A. and Newman, K.E. (2000). The effects of dietary nnanoligosaccharides on cecal parameters and the concentrations of enteric bacteria in he ceca of Salmonella challenged broiler chicks. *Poultry Science* **79**: 205-211.

Uni, Z. and Smirnov, A. (2006). Modulating mucin dynamics using functional carbohydrates. Gut microbiology: research to improve health, immune response and nutrition. *Fifth RRI-INRA Joint Symposium* 21-23 June, Aberdeen, UK.

Wallis, J.W., Aerts, J., Groenen, M.A., Crooijmans, R.P., Layman, D., Graves, T.A., Scheer, D.E., Kremitzki, C., Fedele, M.J., Mudd, N.K., *et al.* (2004) A physical map of the chicken genome *Nature* **432**: 761-764.

The role of nucleotides in improving broiler pre-starter diets

Fernando Rutz, Eduardo Gonçalves Xavier, Marcos Antonio Anciuti, Victor Fernando B. Roll and Patrícia Rossi
Universidade Federal de Pelotas, Pelotas, RS, Brazil

1. Introduction

Environmental management and appropriate nutrition during the first week of broiler life are critical to ensuring optimal performance, despite the fact that the quantity of feed used in this period comprises only 3.5% of total feed intake to market. Yet because neonatal chicks are unable to produce an adult complex of digestive enzymes, digestion is less than optimum (Leeson and Summers, 2005). It is also during these same early days of life that birds face one of their most difficult physiologic transitions: the nutrient sources of lipid and protein in the embryo are replaced by the complex carbohydrates, proteins, and lipids in conventional starter diets. Concomitantly, chick immune systems are immature and chicks are dependent on the antibodies transferred by the breeder (Cutler, 2002).

2. Pre-starter diets

Over the years, broiler body weight gain and feed efficiency have improved, with body weight gain now increasing by a factor of 50 within 40 days of hatch (Noy, 2005). Nevertheless, although chicks grow quite rapidly in the first few days of life, body weight gain can be further enhanced by use of a pre-starter diet (Leeson and Summers, 2005). Based on recent studies on the use of pre-starter feeds to enhance weight gain the following recommendations are offered to improve pre-starter diet effectiveness:

- *Feeding.* Feed diet as soon as possible after hatching to stimulate substrate-dependent enzyme synthesis (Moran, 1990).
- *Quantity.* Offer diet in feeders that are nearly full (Miller, 2005).
- *Metabolisable energy.* Feed intake is governed by both physical satiety and energy intake. Nevertheless, broiler digestive systems do not reach maturity until up to 14 days of age. This delayed maturation may be related to enzymatic development and nutrient utilisation. Therefore, broilers eat to satisfy energy requirements only after two weeks of age (Maiorka *et al.*, 1997).

- *Ingredient quality.* Use high quality ingredients in pre-starter diets. Corn starch is composed of amylose (25%) and amylopectin (75%). Amylopectin has highly branched chains, with greater potential for gelatinisation than amylose. This trait is desirable, because it improves grain digestibility. Collins *et al.* (1999) showed that corn with high amylopectin content (99%) has 2.5% higher metabolisable energy content. Although corn and soybean meal are considered ideal ingredients for broiler chicks during a pre-starter period, Batal and Parsons (2002) observed that diets containing those ingredients had lower metabolisable energy and lower amino acid digestibility than expected in the pre-starter period.
- *Fat.* Chicks have an immature entero-hepatic circulation of bile salts and low lipase synthesis and secretion. Thus, chicks have a lower capacity for digesting fat compared with mature birds. Attempts to add higher levels of fat to the diet may cause oxidation, resulting in destruction of fat-soluble vitamins and damage to intestinal villi. Furthermore, indigestible fat may serve as a substrate for gut microorganisms. Dietary free fatty acids have an adverse effect on fat digestibility (Wiseman and Salvador, 1991), an effect more pronounced for palm oil and tallow than for soybean oil. An absence of dietary monoglycerides also most likely interferes with fat digestibility.
- *Sodium.* Britton (1992) maximised broiler performance by feeding pre-starter diets containing 0.39% sodium. Sodium consumption stimulates water consumption and, consequently, feed intake (Viola, 2003). Furthermore, sodium participates in a secondary active transport system of some nutrients in the gut (Widmaier *et al.*, 2004), a system that is most likely not mature at hatching. Increased dietary sodium content does not cause an increase in litter moisture content. Instead water is retained in the carcass (Vieira *et al.*, 2000).
- *Feed diameter.* Krabbe (2000) evaluated feed mean geometric diameter (437, 635, 780, 866 and 970 μm) of pre-starter diets for broilers and concluded that performance was optimised with diets of mean geometric diameter ranging from 800 to 1000 μm.
- *Protein.* Protein requirement declines as broilers age. Schutte *et al.* (1997) deduced that broiler chicks should not receive a pre-starter diet containing less than 21% crude protein, due to a possible sub-optimal level of glycine and serine. According to Penz (1992), high protein content is necessary in a pre-starter diet. The high heat increment produced by protein plays a role in maintaining body temperature.
- *Additives.* Additives such as enzymes, mannan oligosaccharide, probiotics, and lactic acid (Leeson and Summers, 2005), as well as mycotoxin adsorbents,

antioxidants and mold inhibitors are highly recommended in pre-starter diets.

- *Nucleotides.* Nucleotides are semi-essential nutrients playing a key roles in gut development and repair, skeletal muscle development, heart function and immune response (Grimble and Westwood, 2000). Until recently, it was assumed that all cells were capable of meeting their requirement for nucleotides by *de novo* synthesis. However, recent studies suggest fast growing tissues, such as the intestinal mucosa or tissues related to immunity, along with brain cells and bone marrow, have limited capacity for synthesising nucleotides *de novo* (Yamamoto *et al.*, 1997). To overcome this limitation, those tissues require a supply of nucleotides in excess of what they produce. Those additional requirements can be met by including yeast extracts into the pre-starter diet. NuPro® (Alltech Inc.) is a yeast extract which is rich in nucleotides but also offers other interesting components such as inositol, glutamate, peptides, minerals and vitamins.

3. The effect of NuPro® in pre-starter diets

NuPro® is a high quality nutritional yeast extract derived from a selected strain of yeast. Until recently the use of yeast extracts was destined for human nutrition mainly. As human milk is a particularly rich source of nucleotides, nucleotide supplementation of high quality infant formulas has become an industry standard. Nucleotide enrichment has been shown important for maximising intestinal health. Yeast extract is also used for strengthening the taste of soups, sauces and stocks and as a general taste enhancer. Efficient fermentation technology makes it possible today to use a standardised yeast extract at large in the animal feed industry.

During the manufacturing process yeast is autolysed and components of the cell content such as protein or DNA are hydrolysed and are therefore present in the form of amino acids, short peptides or as nucleotides. Recently much advance has been made to better understand the role of nucleotides on the development of broiler gastrointestinal tract, muscle tissue, and the immune system. Performance benefits have been reported from a series of studies.

3.1. Gastrointestinal development

Feed consumption promotes rapid development of the gastrointestinal tract and associated organs such as liver and pancreas. However, body growth and gastrointestinal tract development do not occur at the same rates. During the posthatch period, the proventriculus, gizzard and small intestine develop faster than overall body weight. Small intestine development is not uniform, with the duodenum growing faster than the jejunum and ileum. The intestines are fully developed between 3 and 8 days of age (Dror *et al.*, 1977). In contrast, the development of lymphoid tissue associated with the intestine parallels increases in body weight consistent with initial feeding rates. At hatch, enterocytes and villi are not well developed and few crypts are present. However, within a few hours posthatch, villi height and area increase rapidly, but not uniformly throughout the intestines. Development is complete at 6 to 8 days in the duodenum and at 10 days in the jejunum and ileum. Crypts increase in number and size, proliferating rapidly during the first days posthatch. Alterations in the enterocytes, villi, and crypts are influenced by diet. For example, delayed feeding of neonatal chicks delays mucosal development (Noy and Sklan, 1997; Uni *et al.*, 1998; Geyra *et al.*, 2001).

The gastrointestinal tract has rapid cell turnover and is unable to produce *de novo* all necessary nucleotides to satisfy its own requirements (Leleiko *et al.*, 1983). Therefore, intestinal development is highly dependent on the presence of dietary nucleotides. Nucleotides increase the development of the villi, intestinal wall thickness, protein content, and DNA and RNA contents (Uauy *et al.*, 1990). Likewise, the synthesis of rRNA in the crypts of the jejunum depends on dietary pyrimidines (Udin *et al.*, 1984). Inflammation in the intestines increases the synthesis of rRNA and consequently, dietary pyrimidine and purine nucleotide requirements (Jain *et al.*, 1997).

Liver weight increases twice as fast as chick body weight during the first week of life (Nir *et al.*, 1993). Endogenous synthesis of nucleotides, mainly in the liver (Mayer *et al.*, 1990), appears to be inadequate to meet nucleotide requirements under conditions of rapid tissue growth and repair or systemic infection. Further, in the case of liver disease, nucleotide requirements increase. The synthesis of hepatic rRNA occurs at a rate of 12 to 25% per day (Grimble and Westwood, 2000). Although the liver is well adapted to supply nucleotides for RNA and DNA synthesis, it is still highly dependent on dietary pyrimidines (Berthold *et al.*, 1995).

Carbohydrates, lipids and proteins are digested and absorbed via an association of pancreatic and brush border enzymes and the presence of intestinal carriers. Posthatch, the activity of intestinal enzymes (i.e., trypsin, amylase and lipase) increases in relation to intestinal weight and body weight (Sklan and Noy,

2000). There is little enzyme secretion between 4 and 14 days posthatch, thus the development of enzymes in the intestinal brush border is highly dependent on the presence of dietary nucleotides (salvage pathway) (Uauy *et al.*, 1990).

3.2. Muscular development

Posthatch muscular development (weight gain) occurs due to hypertrophy of muscle fiber (Widmaier *et al.*, 2004). During this period, cardiac rRNA is synthesised at a rate of 15% per day (Ray *et al.*, 1973). Availability of nutrients after hatch is critical for satellite cell proliferation and for muscular development, thus maximising weight gain. Nucleotides are essential for maintenance and repair of muscle tissue (Grimble and Westwood, 2000).

3.3. Immune system development

Immune system development starts in the embryo and continues post-hatch. During the first week of life, there is a rapid increase in the number of leukocytes, as well as an increase in lymphoid organs (Jull-Madsen *et al.*, 2004). These increases are important for acquired immunity development. Although the yolk sac is important because it transfers passive immunity in the form of immunoglobulins (IgA, IgG) from the yolk and albumen to the neonatal chick (Cutler, 2002), an early excess or deficiency of nutrients can still harm the development of immune response (Klasing, 1998). The synthesis of immune cells is a metabolically expensive process, highly dependent on the presence of dietary nucleotides (Grimble and Westwood, 2000). Macrophage activation and lymphocyte production also depend on nucleotides. Feeding birds NuPro® results in rapid immune system response, as evidenced by increases in lymphocytes and macrophage activity after challenge (Dil and Qureshi, 2002).

3.4. Performance and carcass traits

Basic research suggests that nucleotides are indeed important for optimal development and function of fast growing tissues and thus for optimal performance. Improved performance has been confirmed in different studies. A trial which was conducted at the Federal University of Pelotas in Brazil investigated the effect of dietary NuPro® on broiler performance. A total of 810 day-old male broiler chicks (Ross), housed in floor pens on litter, were assigned to one of nine replicate groups of 30 chicks, three replicates per treatment: (Control) a corn-soybean meal control diet; (Starter +) control diet plus 20 g/kg NuPro®, 1 to 7 days of age; or (Starter-finisher+) control diet plus 20 g/kg NuPro®, 1 to 7 days of age and 38 to 42 days of age. Body weight, feed consumption and feed conversion were evaluated. At trial end, one bird per treatment was euthanised; carcasses were weighed and scored. Birds fed NuPro® from 1 to 7 days of age had higher feed intake and body weight gain than control birds indicating that NuPro® improved performance of broiler chicks when included in a pre-starter diet (Table 1). At trial end, birds fed the supplement in the starter and finisher diet had body weight gain significantly higher than controls and numerically higher than birds supplemented from 1 to 7 days of age only. These findings are consistent with those of Leeson and Summers (2005) who found that, in general, each 1 g increase in 7-day-old body weight improves 49-day-old body weight by 5 g. Birds fed diets containing NuPro® also showed numerically higher carcass yield and yields of drumstick, thigh, wing, and breast weights (not shown).

Improvements in weight gain have been confirmed in a pen trial with male Cobb birds (Figure 1). NuPro® fed from day 1-7 at 2% did significantly improve weight development. This advantage at 7 days grew larger over time, even if all birds received the same diets from day eight onwards. This indicates that optimal early development of the birds will support performance later in production.

Zauk *et al.* (2006) evaluated the performance and carcass traits of broiler chicks fed pre-starter diets (1 to 7 days of age) containing graded levels (0, 1, 2, 3 or 4%) of NuPro®. No significant differences were observed in feed intake, weight gain, or carcass traits. Contrary to results from other studies, this data may indicate differences in the environmental challenge to which birds are exposed

Table 1. Performance of broilers fed diets containing yeast extract (NuPro®).

Treatment	NuPro® (g/kg) 1-7 d	NuPro® (g/kg) 8-37 d	NuPro® (g/kg) 38-42 d	Feed intake (g) 1-7 d	Feed intake (g) 1-42 d	Weight gain (g) 7 d	Weight gain (g) 42 d
Control	0	0	0	162^{b}	4594	83^{b}	2562^{b}
Starter +	20	0	0	177^{a}	4660	104^{a}	2582^{ab}
Starter-finisher +	20	0	20	178^{a}	4626	108^{a}	2631^{a}

^{ab}Means differ P<0.05.

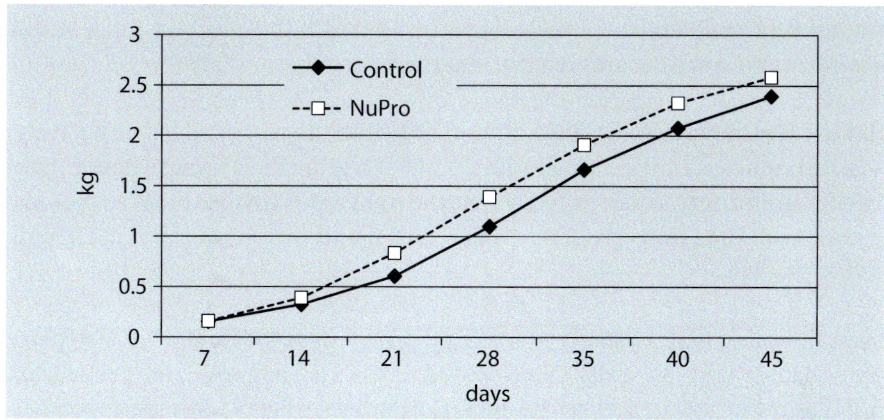

Figure 1. Effect of 2% NuPro® in the starter diets on life performance.

under commercial versus university poultry facility conditions. In contrast, a similar study (0, 1.5, 3.0, 4.5, 6.0 and 7.5% NuPro®) conducted at the Catholic University of Ecuador (Torrealba, personal communication) indicated that weight gain and feed efficiency of both Cobb and Ross strains were significantly increased by inclusion of 1.5% NuPro® in pre-starter diets.

The positive effects of NuPro® on bird performance might become more apparent under stress conditions. In a trial with high bird mortality in the control group NuPro® reduced bird mortality by approximately 30% from 12% down to 8.3% (Table 2). The reduction in mortality can be taken as an indicator for stronger immune defense. In fact several researchers have reported enhanced immune defense with Nupro®. Dil and Qureshi (2002) evaluated the production of leukocytes and macrophage activity in chicks fed diets containing (0, 2.5, 5.0 and 10%) NuPro® and observed improved production of leukocytes and macrophage activity when NuPro® was included up to 5% of the diet. This result

Table 2. Benefits of NuPro in broiler chickens at 42 days of age.

Parameter	Control	NuPro (4%)
Daily weight gain (g)	38.9	39.2
Feed conversion ratio	1.84	1.81
Mortality (%)	12.0	8.3

is consistent with studies in several species in which the effects of nucleotides on the immune system are well documented (Grimble and Westwood, 2000).

There is also indication that the addition of NuPro® does affect flock uniformity. A trial conducted with a 2% inclusion in pullet rearing diets showed better male breeder uniformity. Is seems likely that the number of smaller birds struggling to cope with infectious challenge was reduced and with it overall flock health was improved.

The addition of NuPro® to pre-starter and starter diets for turkey has also been investigated (Table 3). Hulet (2006) tested the inclusion of 4% in the pre-starter and 2% in the starter diet or 3% inclusion in both diets in two performance trials. Hens fed the NuPro® diets had greater body weight ($P<0.05$) at 84 d when compared to the control diet (study 1) and at 95 d in study 2 ($P<0.09$). Although the NuPro®-fed hens had consistently less mortality, no significant difference in mortality or feed conversion was found in either study. The greatest effect appeared to be an increase in feed intake for those hens fed the NuPro® treatments, resulting in increased growth.

Table 3. Effect of NuPro® on performance of turkey hens.

Diet	(n) 1	BW at catch (g)	(n) 1	BW Wk 1 (kg)	BW Wk 3 (kg)	BW Wk 6 (kg)	BW Wk 10 (kg)	BW Wk 12 (kg)
Study 1								
Meat meal	2	59.86	6	0.115	0.558[b]	2.074[b]	5.378[b]	6.840[b]
3% NuPro	2	59.33	6	0.130	0.628[a]	2.259[a]	5.670[a]	7.182[a]
4% NuPro	2	59.64	6	0.128	0.622[a]	2.117[b]	5.598[a]	7.122[a]
P-value		0.6997		0.0597	0.0004	0.0001	0.0001	0.0002
Study 2								
Veg. Protein	2	47.45	6	0.1466[a]	0.6366[a]	2.272[a]	5.859[a]	8.550
Meat meal	2	47.75	6	0.1410[b]	0.6059[b]	2.178	5.727[b]	8.525
4% NP	2	47.33	6	0.1376[b]	0.6096[b]	2.268[a]	5.860[a]	8.733
P-value		0.1766		0.0062	0.0042	0.0027	0.0460	0.0868

4. Conclusion

The fast growing bird requires a high quality pre-starter diet for optimal development. Recent research suggests that nucleotides can improve the quality of pre-starter diets. Nucleotides have been shown to promote chick intestinal maturation and health, brain function, erythrocyte multiplication, hepatic regeneration, skeletal muscle growth and repair, cardiac development, and immune system response. NuPro® supplemented pre-starters have been shown to improve bird quality and performance. Improvements in uniformity are the logical consequence of those changes.

References

Batal, A.B. and Parsons, C.M. (2002). Effects of age on nutrient digestibility in chicks fed different diets. *Poultry Science* **81:** 400-407.

Berthold, H.K., Crain, P.F., Gouni, I., Reeds, P.J. and Klien, P.D. (1995). Evidence for incorporation of intact dietary pyrimidine (but not purine) nucleosides into hepatic RNA. *Proceedings of the National Academy of Sciences USA* **92:** 123-127.

Britton, W.M. (1992). Effect of dietary salt intake on water and feed consumption. *Proceedings of the Georgia Nutrition Conferences Feed Industry,* pp 48-53.

Collins, N.E., Moran, J.R. and Stillborn, H.L. (1999). Waxy corn improves pelleted feed quality, broiler performance and meat yield. *Poultry Science* **78:** 44(abstract).

Cutler, G.J. (2002). Immunity. *In:* Commercial Chicken Meat and Egg Production (Bell, D.D. and Weaver, W.D., Jr., Eds). Springer. New York, NY, USA, pp. 443-449.

Dil, N. and Qureshi, M.A. (2002). Different expression of inducible nitric oxide stnthase is associated with differential Toll- like receptor-4 expression in chicken macrophages from different genetic backgrounds. *Veterinary Immunology and Immunopathology* **84:** 191-207.

Dror, Y., Nir, I. and Nitsan, Z. (1977). The relative growth of internal organs in light and heavy breeds. *British Poultry Science* **18:** 493-496.

Geyra, A., Uni, Z. and Sklan, D. (2001). Enterocyte dynamics and mucosa development in the post-hatch chick. *Poultry Science* **80:** 776-782.

Grimble, G.K. and Westwood, M.R. (2000). Nucleotides. *In:* Nutrition and Immunology: Principles and Practice. Gershwin, M.E., German, J.B., and Keen, D.L., Eds. Humana Press, Totowa, NJ, USA, pp. 135-144.

Hulet, M. (2006). Effect of NuPro on growth performance of turkey hens grown to market age. Poster presented at Alltech's 22nd Annual Symposium, April 24-26, 2006, Lexington, KY.

Jain, R., Malhotra, R., Gondal, Tatke, M., and Vij, J.C. (1997). Nucleolar organizer regions in different colonic epithelia. *Tropical Gastroenterology* **18:** 27-29.

Jull- Nadsen, H.R., Su, G. and Sorensen, P. (2004). Influence of early or late start of first Feeding on growth and immune phenotype of broilers. *British Poultry Science* **45:** 210-222.

Klasing, K.C. (1998). Nutritional modulation of resistance to infectious diseases. *Poultry Science* **77:** 1119-1125.

Krabbe, E.L. (2000). Efeito do peso ao nascer, de niveis e formas de administracao de sodio e do diametrogeometrico medio das particulas sobre o desempenho de frangos de corte ate 21 dias de idade. Tese de Doutorado. Universidade Federal do Rio Grande do Sul. 252 pp.

Leeson, S. and Summers, J.D. (2005). *Commercial Poultry Nutrition.* 3rd ed. University Books, Guelph, Ontario, Canada.

Leleiko, N.S., Bronstein, A.D., Baliga, B.S. and Munro, H.N. (1983). De novo purine nucleotide synthesis in the rat small and large intestine: effect of dietary protein and purines. *Journal of Pediatric Gastroenterology and Nutrition* **2:** 313-319.

Maiorka, A., Lecznieski, J. Bartels, H.A. and Penz, A.M. Jr. (1997). Efeito do nivel energetico da racao sobre o desemphenho de frangoes de corte de 1 a 21 dias de idade. *Anais de Cinferencia APINCO 1997 de Ciencia e Technologia Avicolas. Curitiba.Brasil*, p. 41.

Mayer, D., Natsumeda, Y. and Ikegami, T. (1990). Expression of key enzymes of purine and pyrimidine metabolism in a heptocyte-derived cell line at different phases of the growth cycle. *Journal of Cancer Research and Clinical Oncology* **116:** 215-258.

Miller, S.H. (2005). Keys to brooding management. *Poultry Tribune* **2:** 34-37.

Moran Jr., E.T. (1990). Effect of egg weight, glucose administration at hatch, and delayed access to feed and water on the poult at 2 weeks of age. *Poultry Science* **69:** 1718-1723.

Nir, I., Nitzan, Z., and Mahagna, M. (1993). Comparative growth and development of the digestive organs and of some enzymes in broiler and egg type chicks after hatching. *British Poultry Science* **34:** 523-532.

Noy, Y. (2005). Critical care: early nutrition in poultry. *In:* Nutritional Biotechnology in the Feed and Food Industries, Proceedings of Alltech's 21st Annual Symposium (Lyons, T.P., and Jacques, K.A., Eds.) Nottingham University Press, UK, pp. 35-41.

Noy, Y. and Sklan, D. (1997). Posthatch development in poultry. *The Journal of Applied Poultry Research* **6:** 344-354.

Penz Jr., A.M. (1992). Fundamentos para realizer el cambio de alimento a los 21 dias de edad en pollos de engorde. *Proceedings of XVII Convencion Nacional de ANECA, Puerto Vallarca, Mexico,* pp.232-246.

Ray, A., Mandal, P. and Dessaux, G. (1973). Distribution des acides ribonucleiques dans Le myocarde de rat. Cinetique de marguage par le 32P *in vivo. Archives Internationales de Physiologie de Biochimie et de Biophysique* **81:** 249-272.

Schutte, J.B., Smink, W. and Pack, M. (1997). Requirement of young broiler chicks for glycine+serine. *Archive fur Geflugelkunde* **61:** 43-47.

Sklan, D. and Noy. Y. (2000). Hydrolysis and absorption in the intestines of posthatch chicks. *Poultry Science* **79:** 1306-1310.

Uauy, R., Stringel, G., Thomas, R. and Quan, R. (1990). Effect of dietary nucleosides on growth and maturation of the developing gut in the rat. *Journal of Pediatric Gastroenterology and Nutrition* **10:** 497-503.

Udin, M., Altmann, G.G. and Leblond, C.P. (1984). Radioautography visualization of differences in the pattern of [3H]uridine and [3H]orotic acid incorporation into the RNA of migrating columnar cells in the small intestine. *Journal of Cell Biology* **98:** 1619-1629.

Uni, Z., Ganot, S. and Sklan, D. (1998). Posthatch development of mucosal function in the broiler small intestine. *Poultry Science* **77:** 75-82.

Vieira, S.L., Penz Jr., A.M., Metz, M. and Pophal, S. (2000). Reassessing sodium requirement for the 7-day-old broiler chick. *Poultry Science* **79:** 764-770.

Viola, T. (2003). Influencia de restricao de agua no desempenho de frangoes de corte. 165f. Dissertacao (Mestrado) – Programa de Pos-Graduacao em Zootecnia, *Faculdade de Agronomia, Universidade Federal de Rio Grande do Sul.*

Widmaier, E.P., Raff, H. and Strang, K.T. (2004). *Human Physiology.* 9th ed. McGraw Hill Book Co., Boston, MA, USA.

Wiseman, J. and Salvador, F. (1991). The influence of free fatty acid content and degree of saturation on the apparent metabolizable energy value of fats fed to broilers. *Poultry Science* **70:** 573-582

Yamamoto, S., Wang, M.F., Adjei, A.A. and Amejo, C.K. (1997). Role of nucleotides and nucleosides in the immune system, gut reparation after injury and brain function. *Nutrition* **13:** 372-374.

Zauk, N.H.F., Lopes, D.C.M., Silva, L.M., Dallmann, P.R., Ribeiro, C.L.G., Pinto, A.O., Mielke, R.B., Anciuti M.A. and Rutz, F. (2006). Performance and carcass traits of broilers fed pre-strater diets containing NuPro. *In:* Nutritional Biotechnology in the Feed and Food Industry: Posters presented at Alltech's 22nd Annual Symposium (Suppl. 1). Lexington, KY, USA, p. 10.

Nutrition and gut microbiology: redirecting nutrients from the microbes to the host animal with SSF

James Pierce[1] and Zöe Stevenson[2]
[1]North American Biosciences Center, Alltech Inc., Nicholasville, Kentucky, USA
[2]Alltech Biotechnology Ltd, Dunboyne, Ireland

1. Basic use of enzymes in monogastric feeds

It has become common practice for supplementing pig and poultry diets with enzymes to improve the nutritional value of certain feed materials and positively influence the microflora of the gastrointestinal tract (Table 1). Enzymes act as biological catalysts that, even when present in minute quantities, can initiate and/or accelerate the rate of chemical reactions that transform organic substrates. Digestive enzymes typically act by the process of hydrolysis and thus are classified as hydrolases.

Table 1. Commercial enzymes used in poultry feed: general enzyme classifications relative to substrate specificity and their effects (Adapted from Odetallah, 2005).

Substrate	Enzyme	Effects
Protein Starch Lipids	Protease, Peptidase Amylase Lipase Phospholipase	Supplementation of endogenous enzymes
Phytate (phytin complex w/P, etc.)	Phytase	Enhance plant phosphate use
Hemicellulose (grains) Pentosans (xylose, arabinose) β-glucans Pectins (plant protein sources) Oligosaccharides (mannans, galactans, etc.)	Hemicellulase Pentosanase β-glucanase Pectinase α-galactosidase	Reduction of intestinal viscosity and enhanced nutrient digestibility
Cellulose (plant cell wall)	Cellulase, Cellobiase	Cellulose digestion and release

2. Increasing energy release from carbohydrates

Carbohydrates are the main source of dietary energy in pig and poultry diets and are principally derived from grain. Alternative energy ingredients such as distillers dried grains, wheat middlings and soybean hulls, are also increasingly being used. These types of raw materials are rich in complex carbohydrates, which may influence nutrient availability or absorption and thus interfere with the expected performance of monogastrics at all stages of production.

The major components of cereal grains are polysaccharides, which are macromolecular polymers of monosaccharides linked by glycosidic bonds. The most important of the polysaccharides is starch which is composed of glucose units linked mainly by α-(1,4) bonds as well as α-(1-6) bonds.

Up to ninety-five percent of starch can be digested in the small intestine of birds through endogenous enzyme activity (Geraert *et al.*, 2005). The structure of starch granules affects the rate of digestion and therefore its nutritional value. Starch consists primarily of alpha-glucans in the form of two different polymers, amylose and amylopectin. These two polymers exhibit different structural characteristics which affect their digestibility within the gastrointestinal tract. For example, amylopectin is hydrolysed and absorbed rapidly, whereas the digestion of amylose occurs over a longer period of time (the bonds are not as accessible by digestive enzymes). As a consequence, the digestibility of starch is related to the ratio of amylose to amylopectin. The oligosaccharides stachyose and raffinose can be hydrolysed to glucose and galactose or disaccharides in the proximal small intestine via supplementing the feed with an enzyme mixture containing an oligosaccharidase (Odetallah, 2005).

Non-starch polysaccharides (NSP's) are considered to include celluloses, hemicelluloses, pectins and oligosaccharides (i.e. α–galactosides). The recognition that monogastrics generally do not possess endogenous enzymes to digest the β–linked NSPs has resulted in efforts to develop enzymes that would perform this function. NSPs are associated with plant cell walls and are found mainly in the endosperm of grains but may also occur in the bran. The NSP content varies between different feed ingredients; pearled rice has about 0.8% and sorghum has about 5%, on a dry matter basis (Table 2). Other feed ingredients are generally higher, particularly oats and certain by-products of rice and wheat which may have a NSP content approximating 20-30% of dry matter.

Table 2. NSP content of cereal grains (Adapted from Geraert et al., *2005).*

Cereal grain	NSP (% DM)
Barley	15.9-24.8
Wheat	10.0-13.8
Oat	19.8-38.7
Sorghum	3.4-7.3
Rye	13.2
Triticale	16.3
Corn	8.1
Rice (pearled)	0.8
Rice bran (de-fatted)	21.8
Wheat pollard	35.3

3. Protein digestion

Vegetable proteins such as soybean meal, canola, peas, beans and lupins are all used as the main protein source in poultry diets. Information is limited regarding the effects of indigestible NSPs polysaccharides from vegetable sources. Enzymes with a high level of polygalacturonase activity can depolymerise part of the soluble and insoluble pectic polysaccharides in vegetable proteins. The addition of microbial phytases to hydrolyse plant phytate has proven highly effective in improving phosphorus availability and reducing the anti–nutritive effects of phytate (Touchburn *et al.*, 1999).

The NSP content of vegetable proteins used in poultry diets varies according to their plant origin, the variety, the degree of processing, and subsequently on the proportion of NSP–rich hull in the final product. The total NSP content in vegetable proteins ranges from 180g/kg DM in peas and canola meal to over 350 g/kg DM in some lupin species (Table 3). The major NSP components of the cell wall are pectic polysaccharides which include; rhamnogalacturonan, arabinans, galactans and arabinogalactans (Arora, 1983).

4. Interaction between feed material, NSPs and microflora

The anti-nutritional characteristics of NSPs are numerous, but their effects depend on the specific type of NSP. For example, poultry diets that consist of

Table 3. NSP content of vegetable proteins (Adapted from Geraert et al.*, 2005).*

	NSP (% DM)		
	soluble	insoluble	Total
Soybean meal	6.3	15.4	21.7
Canola meal	1.5	13.9	15.4
Sunflower meal	1.0	19.9	20.9
Lupin angustifolius	3.1	33.6	36.7
Lupin albus	1.4	31.9	33.3
Pea (P. sativum)	5.2	12.9	18.1
Beans (V.faba)	5.0	14.0	19.0
Rapeseed	11.3	34.8	46.1

high levels of indigestible, water-soluble NSPs may predispose birds to outbreaks of necrotic enteritis (NE) (Dahiya *et al.*, 2007). These disease conditions generally occur when diets contain high levels of wheat, rye and oats or barley, as compared to diets rich in corn. The ingestion of high levels of soluble NSP leads to increased digesta viscosity, decreased digesta passage rate and lower nutrient digestibility (Hesselman and Aman, 1986; Choct *et al.*, 1996). Such an effect may decrease nutrient digestibility/availability especially when compared to corn. A highly viscous intestinal environment will increase the proliferation of facultative anaerobes like gram positive cocci and enterobacteria (Vahjen *et al.*, 1998). Larger amounts of undigested material in the small intestine together with a slower flow of digesta increases the chances of rapid bacterial colonisation and in turn creates an environment that can support obligate anaerobes such as *Clostridium perfringens.* It is well documented that the addition of feed enzymes to diets based on wheat, barley, oats or rye significantly decreases viscosity in the small intestine by partially degrading the soluble NSP (Bedford and Classen, 1992; Annison and Choct, 1993). This increases nutrient digestion and digesta flow rate, which reduces the amount of nutrients available to the microflora (Choct *et al.*, 1999). As a consequence the total number of bacteria in the ileum can be reduced by up to 60%.

Due to both the structure of NSPs and the wide range of raw materials they are found in, their adequate hydrolysis and utilisation requires a wide range of enzyme activity (Table 4). Supplementation of diets with an enzyme, or a mixture of enzymes, that are capable of one or more digestive activities

Table 4. Repartition of NSP in the different tissues of the cereal grains (Adapted from Geraert et al., *2005).*

	% NSP				
	Wheat	Corn	Rye	Barley	Rice
Albumen					
Arabinoxylan	65-70	80	60-70	20-30	25-40
Beta glucan	20-30	/	/	65-75	0-20
Cellulose	2-4	/	20	2	30-50
Pericarp					
Heteroxylan	60-65	65-70	/	60-65	55-60
Cellulose	25-30	20-30		25-30	3-9
Lignin	5-10	0.5-1	/	5-10	5-10

improves the energy response to poultry diets. This happens by degradation of specific substrates, which improves the digestibility of feedstuffs in poultry diets (Odetallah, 2005). Endogenous enzymes in poultry are generally specific for α-linked carbohydrates, as are found in starch, so do not generally act on soybean oligosaccharides (raffinose and stachyose) because the α-galactosides cannot be hydrolysed due to the lack of α-1,6-galactosidase activities in the intestinal mucosa.

The upper part of the digestive tract is predominantly colonised by facultative anaerobes, whereas obligate anaerobes are found in the caeca. Beneficial bacteria can protect the gut environment via competitive exclusion of pathogens and are involved in the development of the intestinal immune system. It has been recognised that the modulation of the natural bacterial population of the broiler intestine, through nutritional manipulation such as the selection of feed ingredients or the use of alternate feed supplements, can be an effective tool to control NE. The microfloral population depends very much on the balance between communities of organisms and the diet composition as the source of available substrates for microorganisms. It is therefore unsurprising that a main factor influencing the intestinal microflora is diet composition.

Recently the impact of selected feed enzymes on the digestion (hydrolysis) of non-starch polysaccharides and other non-digestible dietary constituents, has been highlighted. It seems reasonable to assume that non-digestible dietary constituents can be digested, then any additional dietary nutrients provided, will be available to the host animal and gastrointestinal microflora. Non-digestible carbohydrates categorised as oligosaccharides, resistant starch or dietary fibre can particularly affect the composition of the gastrointestinal microflora. They do this by increasing the number of bifidobacteria and lactobacilli (Zentek, 2007). Unpublished data suggests that selected feed enzymes may significantly reduce the incidence of salmonella in corn-based broiler diets and campylobacter in corn and wheat based broiler diets. Based on unpublished data it is also clear that the effect of enzymes on the gastrointestinal microflora is dependant upon the grain source and whether wheat- or corn-based diets are used.

The flora of the gastrointestinal tract principally supports itself by using dietary ingredients as substrates for growth. Depending on the species of bacteria this growth may be either positive or negative. NSPs are not readily digestible within the small intestine of monogastrics due to the absence of required enzyme activities but instead are degraded by bacterial populations in the hindgut. Due to this, NSPs have an effect on gastrointestinal viscosity, which, if increased, seriously impedes nutrient absorption, endogenous secretions, gastric emptying and intestinal transit.

Another class of complex carbohydrates, the α–galacto-oligosaccharides, elicit an unusual physiological response by influencing the availability of metabolisable energy. The undigested oligosaccharides, when present in the lower part of the gastrointestinal tract, are typically fermented by the microflora, producing volatile fatty acids and gases. It is apparent that the extent to which poorly absorbed dietary constituents, such as NSPs and oligosaccharides, are utilised may have a substantial influence on the gastrointestinal bacterial populations and in turn nutrient availability.

5. Comparing types of feed enzymes

Mixtures of enzymes derived from various fungal and bacterial sources and containing a variety of types have been employed against multiple substrates in feed. For some time, most commercial enzyme supplements have been produced using submerged culture fermentations, in which a genetically-modified organism is grown in liquid media and the enzyme produced is separated off. In recent years an 'old' technology, that of solid state fermentation (SSF), has been revived for the production of enzyme complexes for animal feeds. SSF is characterised by the growth of microorganisms on water-insoluble substrates (e.g. wheat bran) in the presence of relatively low amounts of moisture. This system has two advantages; genetically-modified organisms are not needed and using a feed ingredient-type substrate induces a spectrum of enzymes more suitable for the complex nature of animal feeds.

The origin of SSF can be traced back to bread-making methods used in ancient Egypt. Solid state fermentation is also used in a number of well known microbial processes such as composting, silage production, wood rotting and mushroom cultivation. In addition, many familiar western foods such as mould-ripened cheese, bread, sausage and foods of Asian origin including miso, tempeh and soy sauce are produced using SSF. Beverages derived from SSF processes include ontjom in Indonesia, shao-hsing wine and kaoliang (sorghum) liquor in China and sake in Japan (Mudgett, 1986; Table 5).

Solid state fermentation systems provide enzyme activities which are not produced by cultures in liquid fermentation. *In vivo,* feed is not digested by one single enzyme, and it is logical that several enzymes working synergistically can be more effective. For example, phytase enzymes release phosphorus from the phytate complex, but can only do so when the phytate molecule becomes exposed in the cell matrix. Phytate is found most commonly in the cell wall matrix and is usually surrounded by fibrous cell wall material and may also be complexed with starch and protein. In the absence of any side activities, 'pure' phytases are restricted to liberating phosphorus from phytate only when it is exposed or if other enzyme activities are purchased as supplementary enzymes. In contrast, solid-state derived enzymes (e.g. Allzyme SSF, Alltech Inc, USA) also contains several other enzyme activities that can break down fibre (xylanase, cellulase and β-glucanase), crude protein (protease), starch

Table 5. Examples of foods produced by solid substrate fermentation (Adapted from Filer, 2000).

Product	Micro-organism	Materials
Bread dough	*Saccharomyces cerevisiae*	Wheat powder
Cheese	*Penicillium roqueforti*	Wheat powder
Miso	*Aspergillus oryzae*	Soybean, rice
Sake	*Aspergillus oryzae, Aspergillus kawachii*	Rice, barley
Soy sauce	*Aspergillus sojae*	Soybean, wheat
Tempeh	*Rhizopus oligosporus*	Soybean

complexes (amylase) and pectic polysaccharide structures (pectinase). By surrounding and entrapping the phytate molecule, these matrices are disrupted and a greater amount of phytate is exposed to phytase activity (Filer, 2000).

Benefits are gained from hydrolysis of the additional carbohydrate and protein resulting in improved overall performance, as seen in this pig trial (Table 6).

Trials have been carried out to determine the effect of a solid-state derived phytase enzyme on broiler growth rate and phosphorous utilisation in diets typical of those used in Australian broiler production. Live weight gain was improved when Allzyme SSF was incorporated into wheat/soyabean diets containing canola (Figure 1), at both a normal and reduced energy level. A positive effect was also seen in FCR (Figure 2) at both energy levels.

Similar effects have been reported when SSF enzymes were incorporated into corn/soya and wheat/soya diets for broilers (Figures 3 and 4). In terms of weight gain, when Allzyme SSF was added to the reduced energy (-75 kcal/kg) diet, broilers maintained equal performance with the positive control. In wheat soy diets a numerical improvement in weight gain was observed with the low energy diet containing SSF enzyme in comparison to the control diet. Numerically, the best FCR was reported for those birds receiving the low AME and available P diets supplemented with Allzyme SSF.

Table 6. Performance of piglets given a conventional enzyme complement or Allzyme SSF in grower and finisher diets (Taylor-Pickard and Suess, 2007).

	Conventional (200 g/t)	Allzyme® SSF (200 g/t)
Start weight, kg	23.5	23.4
End of grower phase, kg	56.7	54.8
End weight, kg	107.0	113.4
ADG grower, g/day	705	668
ADG finisher, g/day	904	969
ADG whole period, g/day	812	839
FCR grower	2.05	2.12
FCR finisher	2.75	2.50
FCR whole period	2.47	2.37
Carcass weight, kg	84.6	89.6
Lean, killing-out percentage, %	58.3	58.6

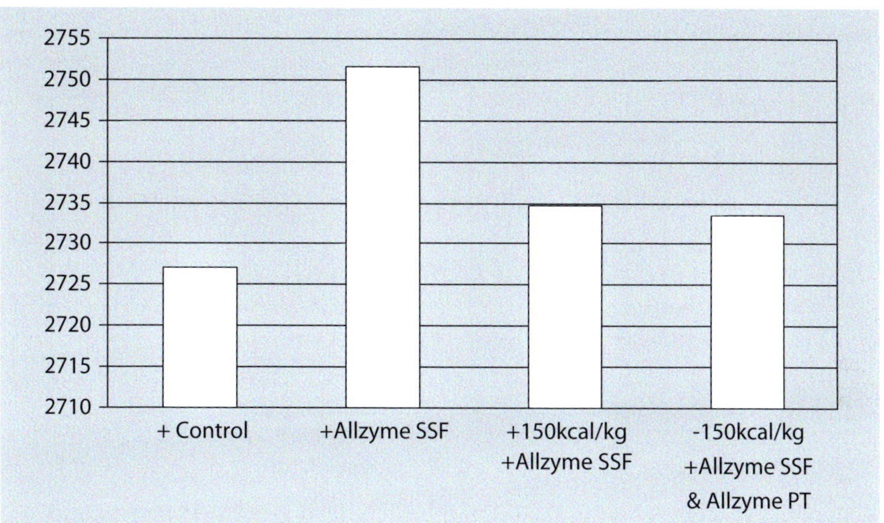

Figure 1. Live weight gain of broilers aged 1 to 42 days fed variable energy diets plus Allzyme SSF (personal communication, Queensland Poultry Research and Development Centre, 2003).

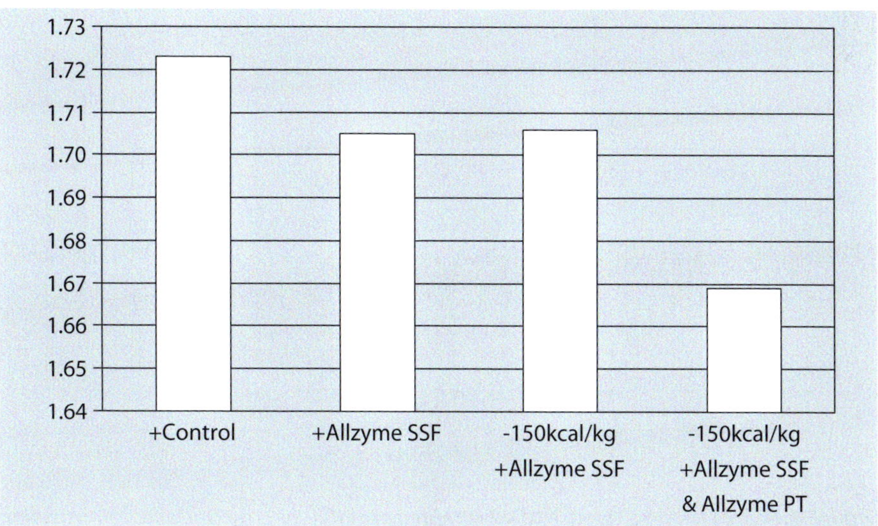

Figure 2. FCR of broilers aged 1 to 42 days fed variable energy diets plus Allzyme SSF (personal communication, Queensland Poultry Research and Development Centre, 2003).

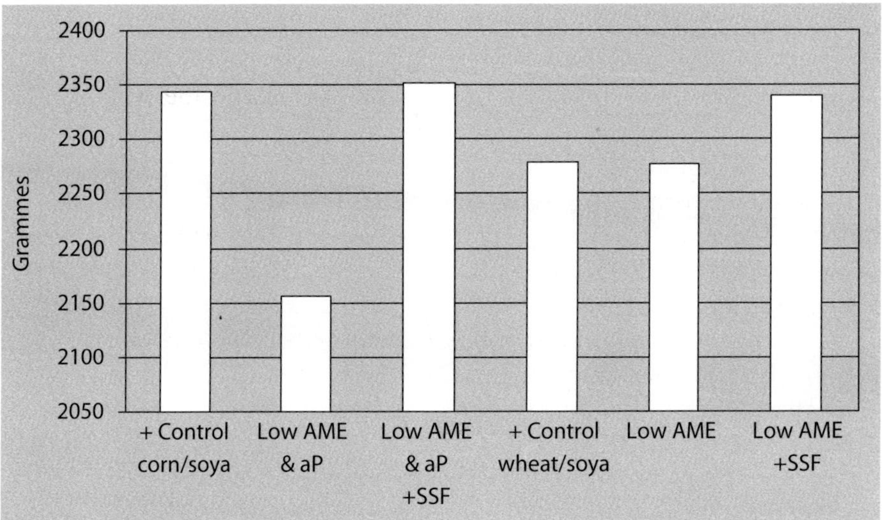

Figure 3. Weight gain of broilers aged 1 to 42 days fed variable energy and phosphorus diets plus Allzyme SSF (personal communication, Queensland Poultry Research and Development Centre, 2003).

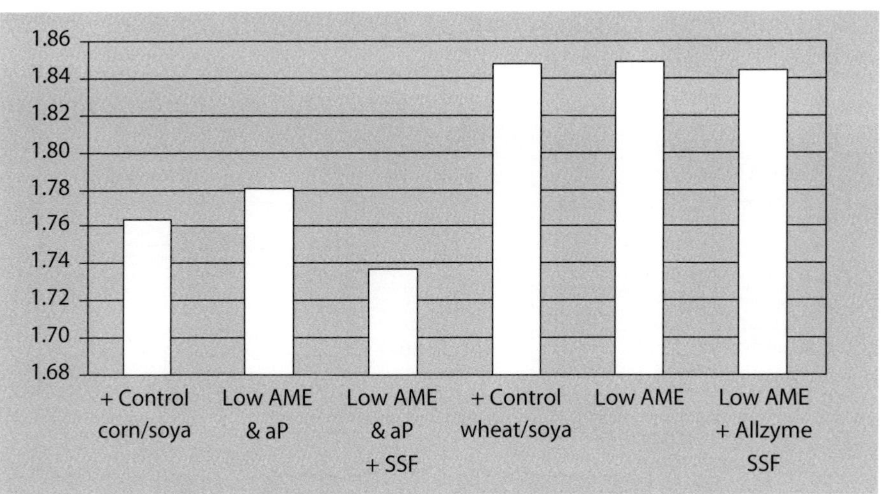

Figure 4. FCR of broilers aged 1 to 42 days fed variable energy and phosphorus diets plus Allzyme SSF (mortality adjusted) (personal communication, Queensland Poultry Research and Development Centre, 2003).

6. Using by-products to reduce feed costs

Due to economic concerns and raw material availability, the typical cereal products used in conventional monogastric diets may be replaced by by-products or low grade feedstuffs which are fibre-rich. In these situations, correct enzyme supplementation is essential if digestion and growth performance is to be maintained. The digestibility of high-fibre or low quality diets poses a problem for most monogastrics. Numerous studies have demonstrated that the digestibility of complex carbohydrates is associated with the chemical structure of such forms of carbohydrates. A case can rather easily be made for the fact that the complex structure of NSPs signals the need for a complex of enzyme activities if the structure of NSPs is to be adequately hydrolysed. The combined action of multiple enzymes assures the desired hydrolysis of divergent categories of NSPs. Disease incidence is also an important consideration as, the colonisation of potential pathogens is greatly reduced in animals fed highly digestible and balanced diets according to their nutrient needs.

7. DDGS a new opportunity or a challenge?

Currently, animal producers are adapting to the use of distillery by-products in the face of rising grain prices, with the shift toward corn for fuel ethanol production in the US and Canada. Similarly in Europe, an impact is forecast from the additional production and demand for grain due to biofuel development. Economics are essentially dictating the use of distillers dried grain solubles (DDG, DDGS, DDS). However, the digestible lysine content can vary among batches or distilleries and practical guidelines for protection against such variation are being sought.

The demand for grain can be estimated using the level of bioethanol production capacity of factories, which is estimated at 7 million tons and is close to estimated bioethanol demand (7.6 million tons) for Europe. Various feed materials will be diverted to produce 7 million tons of bioethanol in 2010-2011, including cereals, sugarbeet, food and non-feed waste, cellulose. Therefore, demand for grain in bioethanol production will reach 17.8 million tons in 2010/11 of which; 4.6 million tons will be for maize, 8.7 million tons for wheat, 1.1 million tons for barley, 2 million tons for rye and 1.3 million tons for other, unspecified grains. Based on increases in animal production, the amount of industrial compound feed manufactured for cattle, poultry and pig should reach 136 million tons by the end of this decade. However, an increase in cereal usage by animals is not likely to follow, because there will be growing competition from rapeseed meal and grain DDGS. It is assumed that the supply of DDGS will reach about 6 million tons and the additional supply of rapeseed meal (due to biodiesel production) will reach 12 million tons at this time. Part of this additional DDGS and rapeseed meal supply is expected to replace cereals in animal diets. DDGS will come from both wheat and maize, the maximum constraint for usage being the large variability in nutritional values.

8. Nutritional value of DDGS

In the dry-mill process, fermentation of grain to produce ethanol essentially removes starch to the greatest possible extent; leaving the protein, fat, fibre, minerals and any other non-fermentable compounds concentrated in the spent grains and liquid solubles. The solubles, which carry the greater part of the fat and minerals as well as substantial amounts of protein, are separated by centrifugation after ethanol recovery. DGGS may have accompanying nutritional problems, including higher levels of mycotoxins, which are not destroyed by the heating of cooking, distillation, and drying. Furthermore, they are concentrated approximately three fold during the ethanol production. On the plus side, DDGS are generally recognised as a good source of available phosphorus. The key issue is knowing how much phosphorus is in any given product. Also, the concentration of these sulphur and sodium can be extremely variable depending on batch-to-batch variations in fermentation, clean out, and the percentage of solubles added to the light grains before drying. Studies have found that total sulphur concentrations range from 200 to over 900 ppm.

The fat content of DDGS is most directly affected by the ratio of grains to solubles. The industry average is around 60:40, and because the solubles contain between 14 and 20% fat and grain contain between 2 and 10% fat, it is easy to understand how the fat levels in DDGS can be so variable. The problem is further compounded by different mixtures ranging from 50:50 to 80:20.

The availability of amino acids in DDGS is directly related to the amount of unused sugar in the solubles and the drying conditions used. Under situations of incomplete fermentation where free glucose remains in the solubles, the free sugars can form insoluble complexes with lysine in a process called a Maillard reaction. Digestible and metabolisable energy levels can be limited due to the variability in the product and the increased fibre concentration compared to grain.

9. Can SSF be used to improve DDGS?

SSF enzyme technology provides a useful strategy to improve the nutritional value of DDGS and addresses some of the concerns associated with feeding this by-product. Enzyme production in SSF systems results in increased amounts of some enzymatic activities not produced by cultures in liquid fermentation. Allzyme SSF also contains activities not found in other commercial enzyme preparations from submerged culture systems (Filer, 2000). Because feed is not digested *in vivo* by one enzyme, it makes sense that several enzymes working in synergy are more effective. *In vitro* comparisons have shown increased rates of reducing sugar, amino nitrogen and an associated increase in phosphate release by an SSF phytase product compared with a pure phytase.

Broiler experiments have been conducted with Allzyme® SSF to examine nutrient release from diets containing 26% DDGS (Pierce *et al.*, 2007). Four treatments were examined in a study with chicks 1-21 days of age; 1. Corn soy reference diet with 22%CP and 3150 Kcal/kg ME, 2. DDGS positive control diet with the same nutrient level as diet 1, 3. DDGS negative control diet with 10% reduction of ME and 5% reduction of CP comparing with diet and 4. Diet 3 + 200 g/T Allzyme® SSF.

The high DDGS diet decreased weight gain and efficiency, which was improved with Allzyme® SSF supplementation (Figure 5).

The trial demonstrated that animal performance could be maintained despite reductions in ME of up to 0.3 MJ/kg in a corn based diet and 0.6 MJ/ kg in a wheat-based diet. The implications with regard to dietary cost savings were significant.

10. Conclusions

Enzymes continue to provide more nutrient release in monogastric diets, contribution the animal growth, feed efficiency and the maintenance of the gut environment and its microfloral populations. With technology available to produce an array of naturally occurring enzymes produced by SSF, we now have an opportunity to get the most energy from conventional diets as well as those formulated with increasingly available by-products, such as DGGS. By improving nutrient availability and digestibility, more nutrients are available

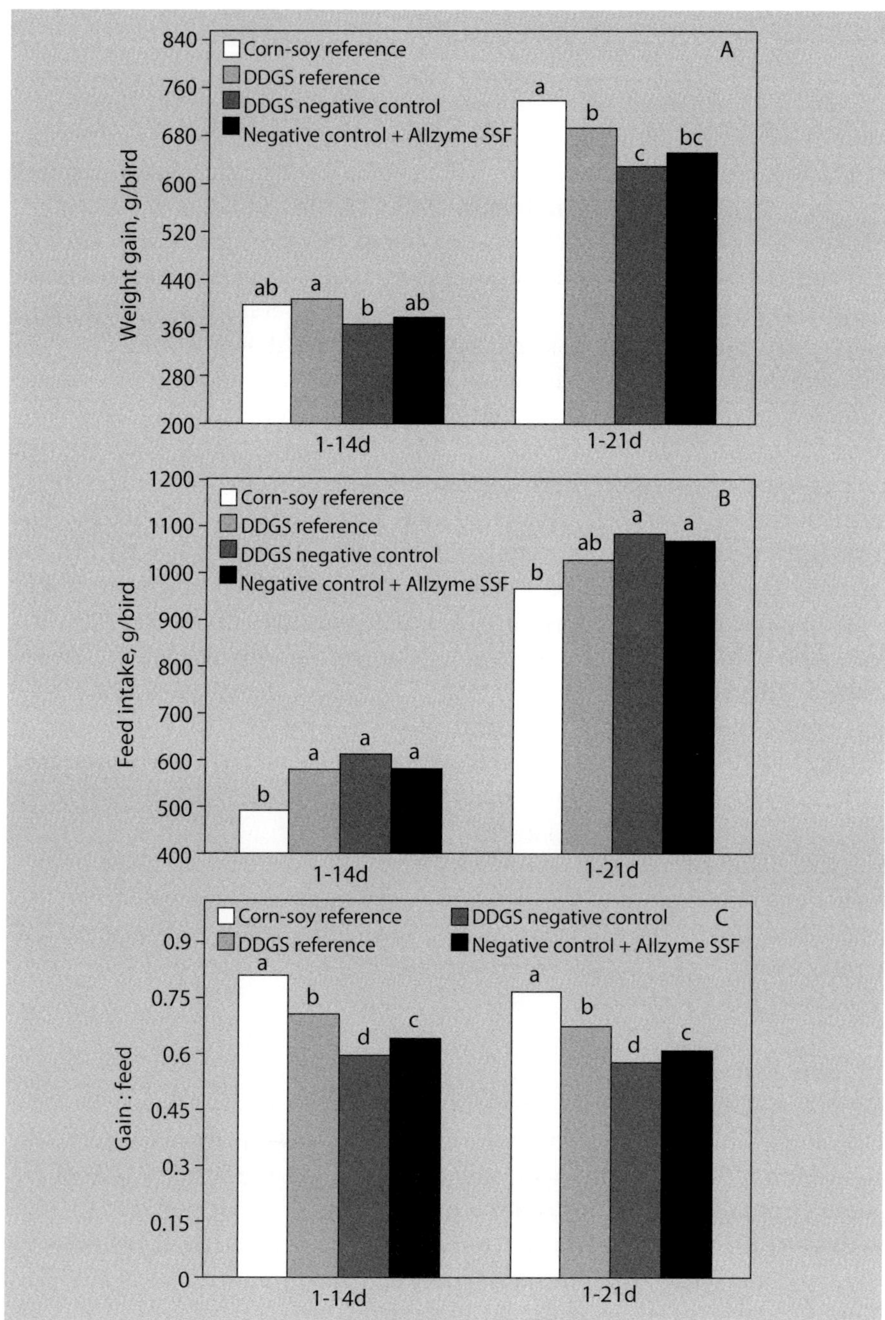

Figure 5. Effect of Allzyme® SSF on weight gain (A), intake (B) and gain: feed ratio (C) of broiler chicks fed diets containing 25% DDGS days 1-21.

for the animal growth and a healthy gut is maintained by reducing the nutrients available to pathogenic bacteria.

References

Annison, G. and Choct, M. (1993). Enzymes in poultry diets. *Proceedings of the 1st Symposium Enzymes In Animal Nutrition*, Kartause Ittingen, Switzerland, pp. 61-68.

Arora, S.K. (1983). Legume carbohydrates. *In Chemistry and Biochemistry of Legumes* (Ed. S.K. Arora). Edward Arnold, London. pp. 1-50.

Bedford, M.R. and Classen, H.L. (1992). Reduction of intestinal viscosity through manipulation of dietary rye and pentosanase concentration is effected through changes in the carbohydrate composition of the intestinal aqueous phase and results in improved growth rate and food conversion efficiency of broiler chicks. *Journal of Nutrition* **122:** 560-569.

Choct, M., Hughes, R.J., Wang, J., Bedford, M., Morgan, A.J. and Annison, G. (1996). Increased small intestinal fermentation is partly responsible for the anti-nutritive activity of non-starch polysaccharides in chickens. *British Poultry Science* **37:** 609-621.

Choct, M., Hughes, R.J. and Bedford, M.R. (1999). Effects of a xylanase on individual bird variation, starch digestion throughout the intestine, and ileal and caecal volatile fatty acid production in chickens fed wheat. *British Poultry Science* **40:** 419-422.

Dahiya, J.P., Drew, M.D. and Haehler, D. (2007). Balanced amino acids control NE: Part 2. *Feedstuffs* **July 9, 2007**, pp. 26-27, 29.

Filer, K., (2000). Production of enzymes for the feed industry using solid substrate fermentation. *In Biotechnology in the Feed Industry, Proceedings of the Alltech's 16th Annual Symposium.* (Eds. T.P. Lyons and K.A. Jacques). Nottingham University Press, UK. pp. 131-151.

Geraert, P.-A., Polais, F., Granier, S. and S. Jakob (2005). Carbohydrates: A review of their physicochemical properties and digestibility in poultry and swine. *In Animal Nutrition Association of Canada 2005 Eastern Nutrition Conference.* pp. 81-82.

Hesselman, K. and Aman, P. (1986). The effect of beta-glucanase on the utilization of starch and nitrogen by broiler chickens fed on barley of low or high viscosity. *Animal feed Science and Technology* **15:** 83-93.

Mudgett, R.E. (1986). Solid-state fermentations. *In Manual of Industrial Microbiology and Biotechnology* (Eds. A.L. Demain and H.A. Solomon). American Society for Microbiology, Washington, DC. pp. 66-83.

Odetallah, N.H., (2005). Enzymes in corn-soybean diets. *In Proceedings of Carolina Nutrition Conference.* pp. 37-49.

Pierce, J.L., Ao, T., Shafer, B.L., Pescatore, A.J., Cantor, A.H. and Ford, M.J. (2007). Effect of Allzyme® SSF on growth performance of broilers receiving diets containing high amounts of distillers dried grains with solubles. International Poultry Scientific Forum, Georgia World Congress Center, Atlanta, Georgia, January 22–23, 2007. pp. 48.

Taylor-Pickard, J. and Suess, B. (2007). Allzyme SSF improves pig performance. *In Nutritional Biotechnology in the Food and Feed Industries* (Eds. T.P. Lyons, K.A. Jacques and J. Hower). Supplement 1: Abstracts of posters presented. pp. 51.

Touchburn, S.P., Sebastian, S. and Chavez, E.R. (1999). Phytase in poultry nutrition. *In Recent Advances in Animal Nutrition* (Eds. P.C. Garnsworthy and J. Wiseman). Nottingham University Press, UK. pp. 147-164.

Vahjen, W., Glaeser, K., Schaefer, K. and Simon, O. (1998). Influence of xylanase-supplemented feed on the development of selected bacterial groups in the intestinal tract of broiler chicks. *Journal of Agricultural Science* **130:** 489-500.

Zentek, J, Hellweg, P. and A. Khol-parisini (2007). Nutritional influence on gut microbial populations. *Nutritional Biotechnology in the Feed and Food Industries* pp. 427-427.

Keyword index

W

Y

Z